LOVE
in the Shadows

LOVE
in the Shadows

Alzheimer's: A carer's story

RHENA TAYLOR

Scripture Union

Scripture Union, 207–209 Queensway, Bletchley, MK2 2EB, England.

© Rhena Taylor 1996

First published 1996

ISBN 1 85999 068 1

British Library Cataloguing in Publication Data
A catalogue record for this book is available from the British Library.

Cover illustration by Rosemary Woods.
Cover design by The Blue Pig Design Company.

Printed and bound in Great Britain by Cox & Wyman Ltd, Reading.

❦ CHAPTER ONE ❦

I suppose that had I known what I know now I would have recognised much earlier the signs of senile dementia in my father; but we are used to passing over the forgetfulness of the old, even our own.

'Did I say Tuesday? Sorry, I really thought I said Thursday. Must be getting old!'

'When did we meet? Nairobi Guest House last June? Sorry, I just don't remember ... Memory going, you know!'

Although we say such things lightly, we don't mean them; and it takes us a long time to accept that something is seriously wrong with the mind of someone we love.

I remember my step-mother, Gwen, saying during one of my missionary 'furloughs' in England, 'I'm worried about your father. I went up to London a week or so ago and left his lunch in the oven. All he had to do was to turn it on, but when I came back in the evening it was still there.'

Dad had always loved his food. It was a family joke in earlier years that he invariably said, 'What a lovely meal, darling!' to my mother after every meal, whether it was baked beans on toast or something she had spent hours on. He must have been hungry at lunchtime that day. Why hadn't he turned the oven on and eaten his lunch?

However, it was something even simpler that brought it home to me.

Gwen was away somewhere and I was cooking. It was mid-summer and I had made a mincemeat tart with custard.

'This is a nice pie. What is it?' he asked.

'It's mincemeat,' I told him. 'I found it at the back of the larder. It must have been left over from Christmas.'

The next day, we ate the other half.

'This is a nice pie,' he said. 'What is it?'

'It's mincemeat!' I said in surprise. 'You asked me that yesterday.'

It was the first time I was to see in his eyes that frustrated annoyance and refusal to comment with which he was to greet any such remark in the early days of this heartbreaking disease. Later, I learnt that the short-term memory is usually the first to go.

Is a fading memory a disease or 'simply' (if that is the word) a consequence of old age? Different points of view are put forward by different people.[1] We are getting used now, in our national media, to the term Alzheimer's, previously applied to younger people who developed dementia. Older adults were said to suffer from 'senile dementia' (giving rise recently to that frightening term 'dements'). Doctors and scientists continue to disagree about the separation of the two terms. One point about which there is no disagreement, however, is the increase in numbers of those affected by the condition. Whichever term we use, we are going to hear more and more about it in an ageing population where it is estimated that, by the year 2011, one million people will suffer from it.

It seemed the symptoms of 'whatever it was' came

slowly to my father. There were the slips of memory (nearly always the short-term variety) that were disquieting, but we tried to forget them. He was in his own house in a quiet Norfolk village, following a routine he was happy with and his beloved wife at hand. There was little to upset or worry him. Even after these first signs of a failing memory I continued to work in Kenya, although I began to take 'local leave' in England which meant I returned for a month every year.

Each time I came, differences were apparent. Gwen was unwilling to leave him alone overnight and, when I came home, she naturally took the opportunity to visit her sisters in London for a few days. Her departure clearly unsettled him. I had a desk in my room and work to do. After lunch, when he was used to sitting quietly with Gwen and the newspaper (which he had almost ceased to read although he liked it near him) and was dropping off to sleep for a time, I used to go upstairs and try to catch up with whatever letter or article I was writing. But he was unhappy at being alone and was clearly dozing off and waking frequently. When he woke, he did not know if anyone was in the house or not. So, slowly because he was walking with difficulty by that time, he would stump up the stairs and shuffle along the corridor to my room. Thump, thump, thump. Shuffle. Shuffle. Then the door would be pushed open.

'Oh, hello, darling. You're here, are you? Are you all right?'

'I'm fine, Dad!' I would answer. 'Would you like to sit here with me for a bit?'

'No ... No, I'm all right. Just wanted to know where you were.'

A receding thump, thump, thump.

Ten minutes later I'd hear the chair being pushed back in the dining room and the whole thing would start again. And again. And again.

We loved my father – Gwen and I. Looking back, I know he was fortunate to have two people who loved him and who were able to care for him through his last years. And we were lucky to have had each other. I view with disbelieving dismay recently published statistics which estimate that 154,000 people with dementia live alone in the UK.[2] However, Gwen and I would have had to be saints if we had never got irritated sometimes!

I suppose it would have been a small thing for me to have given up working on my article and gone down to sit with my father when Gwen was away. But then it was my life too. I'm not the kind of person to sit and sleep through an afternoon, and at the time I was still trying to pretend that life was normal. In fact, I usually stuck it out for a time – telling myself the doctor had said exercise was good for him! – and then went downstairs and tried to continue writing by hand at the dining room table. Unfortunately, by then I was totally enslaved to using a computer so that little work was done on those afternoons.

Then the 'Where's Gwen?' syndrome started whenever she was out of sight. Whether she was in the next room or away in London, he would ask, 'Where's Gwen?' every ten minutes or so.

'Where's Gwen?'

'She's visiting her sisters in London.'

'When is she coming back?'

'On Friday.'

'Oh. That's nice.'

A slight pause. Then…
'Where's Gwen?'
What made one feel worse was that Dad was entirely courteous. It was impossible to feel angry at him, only at ourselves for experiencing the kind of irritation we did. I know (now) that 'carers' (a term I only heard after a year or so in England) must fight the feelings of guilt about this. At the same time, I do think that annoyance and irritation in the carer greatly contribute to the unease and unhappiness of a person whose mind is gradually slipping away.

'Oh, don't mind him,' a wife said to me once, when her husband had addressed some incomprehensible remark to me as I dished out meals on wheels. 'Silly old fool!'

Her comment hurt me, even if it was her way of trying to pretend to herself and to me that it was just 'silliness' that made him like this. What efforts we make to pretend it isn't really happening, that it isn't getting worse.

What, after all, is 'it'? Before we got involved I knew little or nothing about senile dementia and had never heard the word Alzheimer's. Even when we became caught up in a situation that involved the disease, I still knew very little; but it was the last thing I wanted to read or talk about. Neither Gwen nor I, as things got worse, felt a desire to go to any 'support group' or read any articles or books on the subject. The present situation facing us was all we could manage, day by day.

Of course, there were two of us when I finally came home from Kenya, although Gwen had managed the earlier years alone. Quite honestly, I think had I been alone in those later years I could neither have written nor spoken about them now. Being one remove from it made me retain just enough objectivity to be able now to share with others the experience of living through the darkness of dementia with someone I loved.

One tried all sorts of things. In the 'Where's Gwen?' period I once wrote in big letters 'GWEN IS AT THE HAIRDRESSER' and put it on the mantelpiece.

'Now, if you want to know where Gwen is, just look there,' I told father. But he just got up, with an annoyed expression, and crumpled the paper in his hand.

I wonder how much he knew in those early years. He never told us his thoughts. I remember a woman saying to me that she watched her mother weeping for hours because she knew she was losing her mind. But for father, he drew the curtain back just once or twice.

'It's like water suddenly running through my mind,' he said once when we were alone. 'Sweeping everything away...'

'Never mind, darling. It doesn't matter. I'm here,' I said.

Then there was the question of shutting the garage door. We live in a village where security is not a very high priority. However, the overhanging garage door led straight into the back garden and we generally shut it from the outside at night. Father clearly used to do that as one of his night chores, but now every night he could not remember whether he had shut it or not.

'Where are you going?' we would ask as he struggled to his feet while we were watching television, and shuffled towards the front door.

'To shut the garage,' he would reply.

'But it's shut.'

He would still go out into the night, returning in a moment without comment. The only way we could cope was to let him do it again and again until he finally became too tired or forgot about it.

I met a friend in Bristol during this period, who had gone through this with her mother.

'You're lucky,' she said to me. 'My mother had the same conviction that we had not shut the garage door, but she insisted I get up and see that it was shut – every five minutes or so.'

What stories lie behind the experiences of people caring for those with dementia! Few can tell them.

Things were clearly worsening and Gwen, herself nearing 80, could not be left much longer to manage alone. I returned once more to Kenya, this time with the intention of leaving for good at the end of the following year.

Today, the term 'carer' is in common use. There are said to be nearly 7 million carers in the UK, that is people looking after relatives or friends who, because of disability, illness, or old age, cannot manage at home without help. On the whole, it remains an acknowledged maxim in Western society that the old should be cared for by younger members of the family clan; but when, where and how are debatable.

'My father's in a London home,' said one lady in Bedford to me.

'Is he happy there?' I asked.

'No. He hates it. We can't take him gifts because the nurses take them from him as soon as we've gone. He cries when we leave.'

I've never forgotten that. 'How could she?' I cried inside. If it had been me, I would have done anything to have brought someone I loved out of such a situation. But then it wasn't me. Perhaps she *didn't* love him that much. Maybe there were childhood hurts she had suffered at his hands. Perhaps she felt she would lose her husband if she insisted her father came to live with them; or alienate her children. But I couldn't stop the thought: if that had been a Romanian baby whom she could have adopted, would she have left him there crying when she went?

But it was her decision before God, as it is yours and mine.

There was another issue involved in my coming back from Kenya at that particular time. I believed God was calling me into a new ministry in the UK – evangelism among the old.

Perhaps it was the 'African blood' in me that caused me to see the marginalisation and often outright unhappiness of older people in the West. Who was concerned to take the message of the gospel to the old in our increasingly ageing population? I had started speaking and writing about this ministry in 1986, at first looking to organisations already in existence to take this speciality in tow. But – as so often happens when we identify a need – by September 1987 I had accepted that, after twenty-eight years in Africa, I was being called by God to my own country to bring this ministry into being. I shared this with the General Secretary of my mission, and in May 1988 sent out my first letter to friends to 'float' the idea. A recently retired pensioner in the West Country sent me five pounds. I looked at it in my Nairobi flat – the first gift for a new ministry. Since then I have received over £40,000; but I will never forget that five pounds. Who shall despise the day of 'small things'?

I had a call, a vision, and I had an ailing father. The two things together made my departure from Kenya perfectly understandable on all sides. Quite apart from their strong sense of family responsibilities, many Africans in their fifties start looking to their 'home areas' and seek to do good there. It all fell into line. I left in peace, with an African prayer letter list of over seventy people committed to praying for me in England. I am still looking forward to doing 'deputation' (now called 'mission education'!) in Kenya.

NOTES

1 These are often summarised and documented by the Alzheimer's Disease Society's monthly newsletter (available from Gordon House, 10 Greencoat Place, London SW1P 1PH).
2 *Home Alone*, published by the Alzheimer's Disease Society (July 1994).

❧ CHAPTER TWO ❧

I said goodbye to my African life and friends. I was 55. From being a communication officer for an African Archbishop – a job that had been continually interesting and challenging – and from other media commitments that had taken me to widely different parts of Africa, I became a 'carer' (only later learning to use that term) in my parents' house in a small Norfolk village. I had the two trunks I brought from Africa carried to one of the outhouses and did not try to unpack them.

'Hello, darling,' my father said when I came into the room. I knew he did not know whether I had come back from Africa after a year or from Swaffham after an hour, but his welcome was real.

Gwen and I were babes as far as nursing went or as far as understanding or using the NHS services available. Cancer in the anal area had been diagnosed some years previously, and this caused father to be partially incontinent; we had to look for some kind of padding. When I arrived, Gwen was trying to make something of cotton wool, and I went shopping in Boots, ending up buying some babies' disposable nappies. It was only some months later that one of the assistants in Boots kindly introduced me to the world of incontinence pads. Much later, we discovered we could get them free on the National Health. We became experts in them as time went on, calling them the yellow (light), green (medium), and blue (highly absorbent). I could have kept a dinner-table conversation going for hours on their particular facets. ('Do you realise that the highly absorbent incontinent pads are said to be able to hold eight pints of liquid?'!) Perhaps it's as well there weren't that many dinner invitations around in a Norfolk village.

Neither of us 'minded' that kind of nursing, although, had I been asked previously, I would have said it revolted me. In fact, both Gwen and I had a highly developed sense of humour which stood us in good stead throughout. It was no good getting upset about accidents: such as when I put a bright red towel into the washing machine and turned all father's underpants pink. At least it ensured, when he later had times of 'respite care' in hospital, that we got his spare underpants back.

In those early days life was reasonably normal. Father could still be left for short periods in the day-time and we could take turns being away at night. Although I missed my African friends, I did appreciate being back in England for many reasons and very much had my mind on the vision God had given me. I attended various conferences and visited friends when I could. Gwen could also visit her son and family in Kent and London. But there was still the consciousness that father was really not with us now and that we were gradually saying goodbye. Our thoughts became more and more centred on him.

People call Alzheimer's Disease the 'long bereavement', and I understand this term now. In body the one you love is still there; but he or she is no longer fully there. Gwen had known this for some time. Previously she and father had both taken a keen interest in politics and enjoyed a lot of discussions on topics arising from the morning paper or the radio. Now father could not really hold a long conversation, although he was still capable of making sudden, surprisingly intelligent remarks about what we were saying. However, for Gwen to sit there every morning with him, as she had done for over twenty years, and not be able to talk with him intelligently was one of the hardest things for her to bear – and I was not a very good substitute.

Communication powers go quite soon with Alzheimer's Disease. I had known for some years previously that I could no longer discuss my situation or any personal problem I might have with father. He would try, but lose the thread very soon.

It was the same with television. Gwen and I both liked good films and would happily sit through one in the evening. Father would fairly often interrupt.

'It's silly, isn't it?' he would say.

'No, it's not,' I would say. 'We're enjoying it.'

He would accept that, but some minutes later he would say again, 'Isn't this silly?'

Sometimes he would initiate a conversation quite suddenly with no warning, perhaps while dozing after lunch.

'Has … that man … come yet?'

We would both welcome it.

'What man, darling?' Gwen would say. 'Did you see someone through the window?'

'No … It was just that … Well, you know, he came before … I was going to … Oh never mind!'

This closed most such conversations, '… Oh, never

mind!' The programme could not finish.

Short, easy responses he could manage. I never once put a cup of tea beside him when he didn't say, 'Thank you, dear.'

When we passed him sitting in his chair, he would say, 'Don't work so hard. Come and sit down.'

No one came into the room that he did not greet with, 'Oh ... Hello. Do sit down.' In fact, visitors used to wonder what we were finding so difficult. He looked the same as anyone else – well and healthy for a man of over 90. The cancer he was suffering from grew slowly and did not appear to give him pain. Only we knew his mind was continually wandering somewhere else, somewhere we could not follow: a world of changing shadows, shafts of sudden light that only too soon died away in the half-darkness of the 'somewhere else.'

Somewhere inside he was still there, the real person. Something was telling him he should not inconvenience us by asking us to 'shut the garage', and should do it himself. His mannerisms, his courtesy and consideration, his love of a good meal: they still identified him as the husband and father we knew and loved.

We learned not to worry about trying to follow the conversation. Since then I have seen frustrated visitors in a nursing home: 'But I'm Mrs Wilson from down the street! You remember, don't you? Mary Wilson! I used to take you shopping...' The voice would get louder as the speaker tried to help the older person to remember them rightly.

I wonder why it is so important to be recognised? If a train is running quietly along one track, why force it into another? Just get into the one that's running.

'Have you found them?' father would say suddenly.

'Found what, dear?'

'Oh … you know, those books…'

I have no memory of losing books or talking about them. But I know unexpected cross-files can turn up on the computer screen…

'Oh, yes. I found them yesterday.'

'Where were they?'

'Under the table in the hall.'

'Oh. That's good.'

He is quiet and satisfied.

I felt no guilt from that kind of conversation. I was not mocking him or laughing at him. I was helping him resolve that little piece of the jigsaw and lay it quietly down. To try and get him to identify *which* books and *when* we had 'lost' them, if we had, would only have resulted in the frustrated 'Oh … You know … Never mind!'

Laughter at such wandering minds is, to my mind, totally inappropriate.

I had a dearly-loved aunt who told me once about her older neighbour who had cut out pictures of Charles and Diana (soon after the wedding) and put them in different armchairs and 'had them to tea'. When my aunt knocked on the door, she was told, 'Shh! You'll have to wait until they've gone.'

'Laugh!' my aunt said. 'I was in stitches!'

I said nothing but I was hurt for her neighbour. A wandering mind is no subject for laughter, any more than any other part of the body which is malfunctioning. But I recognised that part of that laughter was due to my aunt's own unexpressed fears: 'I'm old now. What if it were me? But it isn't. Look! I can find it funny!'

Gwen and I learned – or tried to learn – that raising our voices was unhelpful. When we said something to father there was sometimes no reaction at all, and the natural response was to repeat what we had said in a louder voice.

'Don't shout!' he would say in irritation.

We realised later that it wasn't a case of not having heard us, more a case of unjumbling the sounds into something meaningful.

Time was a problem too.

Father would suddenly decide we needed potatoes and go to the shop for them. Fortunately, the shop was only just down the street and across the road. He went once (in the summer) at about 9.30 pm and I met him coming back,

'It's shut!' he said in amazement.

Another time I went to the loo at about 5 am in the summer months and put my head around the parents' door, just to check. Gwen was dozing and father was not there.

I looked in the bathroom and the other bedroom. Gwen started up: 'What's the matter?'

'Where's father?'

'I thought he went to the loo...'

We found him in his pyjamas downstairs in the sitting-room, shivering and wet.

'Where is everyone?' he said pathetically.

I know wandering is one of the most difficult facets of this disease but, apart from the relatively rare situation mentioned above, father did not worry us like that. As I have said, he was in totally familiar surroundings and always loved his home anyway. He was now rarely left alone – for as his world was shrinking, ours also was becoming more confined.

Some years earlier father had developed sight problems and Gwen took over the driving for them both. One of their pleasures had been quiet, leisurely drives to Blakeney or Sheringham, where they would walk along the coast a little way and have a meal or coffee in a country pub. Now being driven anywhere made him nervous.

'Where are we going?' he would ask continually. 'Can we go home now?'

Once I remember driving him with Gwen to Cromer and stopping the car at the top of the cliff overlooking the sea. When we arrived somewhere father seemed to accept it, and how he had always loved the sea. He walked a little way with us, then stood holding onto my arm looking along the cliffs and out to the distant haze of sun and sea. I knew he was saying goodbye. I had seen it once before in Mombasa. He and Gwen had visited me in Kenya in 1980, his eightieth year. We had gone to Mombasa and were on the way to catch the train back to Nairobi. It was near the end of their stay. He was standing looking out across the blue Indian Ocean broken by the line of white waves over the coral reef and to the shoreline of palm trees outlined against an evening sky.

'It's time to go,' I said. 'What are you doing?'

'Saying goodbye to all this,' he said. 'We'll never see it again.'

The same look was in his eyes now. He knew he would never see the sea again.

What of those who grow old, whose sight fails, whose disability means they will never again walk along cliffs and smell the salt wind or hear the sound of the breakers? What of my father who would never again look out across the sea he loved? Is this old age? Loss. Giving up. For ever?

I cannot believe that God gives us beautiful things and a love for them, only to take them away. I want to believe that in heaven there will be these same familiar things – more beautiful than ever. A new heaven and a new earth...

Then there was his wine-making equipment. Father had long enjoyed wine-making. Gwen and I and anyone else visiting would often be cajoled into picking blackberries along the roadside on in an old airfield near us. Father could outpick all of us easily. Then there were elderberries and, when these failed, he would go to the market and come back with sacks of cheap oranges. Now there were vats 'processing' in the linen cupboard, and dozens of bottles outside in the shed waiting to be filled, as well as all the other equipment he needed. The latter could be given away but I had no idea what I should do with the vats. Gwen, usually very good about sentimental things, found this one rather hard – after all, they represented a lot of work. In the end, on a day when she was out, I poured the liquid away and left the empty vats in the shed to give to anyone who wanted them. It was the end of something else that had been happy.

Saying goodbye. We all have to do it as life draws towards its end. St Paul says, 'If for this life only we have hope in Christ, we are of all men most to be pitied' (1 Corinthians 15:19). I believed father to be a Christian. He and my mother had both been children of missionaries in China where I and my brother had been born. Neither were especially 'active' in their faith, but they were intermittent churchgoers and never hostile to Christian things. Earlier, as I saw father grow older, I had asked him, 'What if you die, Dad? Do you believe you'll go to heaven?'

He had looked at me and answered quietly, 'You know, Rhena. When children go to a father, there is nothing to be frightened of. You know you'll be welcomed.'

I have often thought of this since. Something in me wanted to say, 'But, Dad, have you really understood what being a Christian is? Have you committed your life to Jesus?'

But I didn't. It seemed enough to me. I have always remembered the woman with an 'issue of blood' in Matthew 9:20–22. All she did was touch the hem of Jesus' garment, and it was enough for Jesus to say, 'Your faith has saved you. Go in peace.'

❧ CHAPTER THREE ❧

Before I lived with my father in his closing years, my attitude to the mentally disturbed was probably one of fear and unease. I remember reading Salinger's *Catcher in the Rye* when I was at University and being very willing to take it back to the library! The vivid insight into a slipping mind was too real, too frightening.

Yet, when I became accustomed to living with my father, I found this attitude quite hard to forgive in others.

A vicar in north London once told me that an old woman from the neighbourhood had knocked on his front door at about 9 pm on a weekday evening, asking why the church lights were not on as it was time for evensong.

'What did you do?' I asked.

'I got my wife to go for one of her neighbours,' he said. 'I just can't handle that kind of thing.'

'Why not?' I thought to myself. 'It is only an illness, like anything else.'

I had come a long way in a short time.

This inability to face up to dementia is clearly stated in a report from the Board of Social Responsibility for the Church of England published in 1990:[1]

Many of those who tend people with dementia find that in order to survive they must distance themselves from the most acute distress. This distancing may be both emotional, caring being reduced to the purely physical since the 'real' person is felt to have died some time before, and geographical, the sufferer being taken into residential care. It has been observed that nursing staff may place those most severely affected furthest from their office and the entrance to the ward, and the visiting clergy may spend most of their time with patients most capable of dialogue. Distancing leads easily to denial. Clergy omit to mention dementia in funeral services, hospital doctors refuse to admit that there is a need for increased provision, services for people with dementia are underfunded compared with acute services. Sufferers are made to disappear into 'the community' or isolated mental hospitals and frequently we think 'it would be better if s/he died'. While we may have begun to confront our fears about cancer or AIDS, dementia leaves us overwhelmed.

We were, as I said, in a village. Had father been suffering from something else, I'm sure neighbours would have offered to keep an eye on him occasionally, even perhaps for a day or two while we took a break. But as it was, the more honest among them said something like, 'I'd love to stay with him, Rhena. But I'm frightened of what he'll do.'

As things got more difficult, we gradually learned what the NHS could and would do, and discovered other voluntary organisations who were willing to come in and sit with father to give us a break. I suspect that these were a little easier to contact because father had cancer as well as dementia. We discovered that at least one very good organisation was there to support cancer sufferers only.

The difficulty, especially in the early days, was to be honest enough to say what kind of help we really needed. Both Gwen and I were the kind of people to accept any sort of help with immense gratitude; yet being very unwilling to ask for anything special.

For example, it was 'agreed' that Jean would come on Tuesday and Thursday afternoons so that Gwen and I could go out for a while. Gwen, by now, was really too tired and upset to drive herself anywhere unless I went with her. But where to go? Shopping in Swaffham did not hold much charm. We were fifteen to twenty miles from any other town and (when this kind of help first started) it was the holiday season and the roads were hot and busy. Anywhere we went cost money – stopping for tea, visiting a National Trust place – and we ended up worried about getting home at the right time for Jean because we were being held up in the holiday traffic.

We had both friends and relations within thirty miles. Visiting them was good but not always convenient. Our 'sitters' came when they could (and we were grateful) but lunchtime, for instance, was not always the best time to visit my aunt who was in a residential home in Fakenham. If we did have lunch with friends, we had to rush back afterwards.

After some months, however, we came into contact with one official of the 'Home Hospice' group, who accurately saw what both Gwen and I needed and provided it. I needed time to myself and more 'space'; Gwen needed physical and mental rest without the constant alertness to father's movements. So Margaret came at least once a week and took Gwen out with her, either visiting or perhaps to her own home where she could lie back and relax, leaving me in the house alone with father who, by now, slept a lot of the afternoon. It gave me the space and quietness I needed and Gwen the rest. Later, the same carer was instrumental in helping us to get 'respite care', where for a time father was looked after in a nearby cottage hospital for one week in six. This really gave us the best kind of relaxation – to be at home and not on the alert – and also made it possible to go away for a few nights. For me, still with my future on my mind, these breaks were vital, giving me a chance to remember I still had a future.

Another helper we remember is Maureen, a large and cheerful 'bath attendant'. Father had loved his daily bath, but it had got more and more difficult to help him out of it once he was in. We tried so many different things, but by now anything unfamiliar was confusing. A bath shower was resisted and the bath seats we tried were just not workable.

'There's something there!' he would say as we, having got him standing in the bath, tried to encourage him to sit down on the seat. Despite our pleas and attempts at explanation, as soon as his bottom touched the unfamiliar object he would struggle to stand up again, his legs and arms trembling with the effort. When we had to call in a neighbour to help us lift him out of the bath one day, we had to give up the idea of a regular bath and Maureen arrived on the scene to give a 'blanket bath' twice a week.

Kind, loving and considerate as father was, as dementia took hold, he could grow very angry at being 'forced' to do anything. I had never known him to swear, but now he would frequently hit out and push people away, 'Get the hell out of here!' he would say angrily. 'Leave me ALONE!'

But Maureen was always cheerful. 'Come along, sweetheart,' she used to say. 'Won't take long.'

Then we would share a cup of coffee afterwards, while father lay, clean and with his hair brushed neatly, looking like a frustrated small boy who had just had to wash behind his ears. We appreciated this kind of professional help very much.

Trying to explain things to other family members, however, was difficult. My brother, Don, lived at a distance and had a family of five. When he visited, he could not really accept the fact that father looked as usual but was not.

In one visit Don said something about Jane (the oldest grandchild) who had been accepted for a job.

'Jane?' said father. 'Who's Jane?'

This upset Don. Surely he should remember his first grandchild? In the beginning Don saw it as indifference, an indication that father no longer cared about the children, and it hurt him. It was so hard to explain that father no longer held such things in his memory and that it was not a matter for blame or for hurt feelings.

'Where are you going?' he asked Don on another occasion as he got up to go.

'I have to go home,' Don told him. 'To Southampton.'

'Southampton?' father said. 'That's a silly place to live.'

For Don this was hard, and he was struggling with anger.

'What kind of remark is that?' he said to me on the way out.

I have since heard others speak of very upsetting and hurtful things said by those with dementia. It seems certain words recur in the brain and are used. Father never (as I remember) used the word 'silly' much in his normal life. Why now? I had long stopped worrying about what was said, but I realised his words still had the power to hurt those who saw him physically as he ever was and could see no outward sign of what was happening to him. We 'worked' quite hard to prepare father for meeting different relatives.

'Dad, your nephew's coming today. Arthur. You know – Arthur and Johnnie. You remember them, don't you? They live in Norwich. They're coming to visit you...' and so on, trying to cushion the blow for those who would find it hard to realise his fading mind.

Later, at the funeral, Don said to me, 'I had said goodbye a long time ago.'

The long bereavement.

As our world closed in on us, friends at a distance became more and more unreal. Sometimes they phoned, even came to visit if they were passing. But it was difficult. Was the bathroom clean for them? Where and when could we talk? We could not leave father alone for long periods, and it was hard to talk simply as if he wasn't there. How about getting his meals and helping him eat them? How about leaping up every time he wanted to go to the loo, and the disturbed nights? On the whole, we did not encourage house visitors much. 'Keep up your relationships,' I remember hearing from one advisor, but it is easier said than done. One does not have much emotional energy left.

As someone trying to keep at least a memory open in the working world, I could not but notice the attitude of other professional people to me at this time. I remember one such person meeting me in London to find out more about the vision God had given me for reaching older people with the gospel. She was enthusiastic, ready to go into ways of how what she was doing would fit into what I was doing, ready to make plans.

Then she found out I was a 'carer', committed to my father.

'So you're not free,' she said flatly.

'Not right now,' I agreed. 'But I believe the time will come soon when God will...'

'Others say that,' she said, interrupting me but speaking almost to herself. 'Things like that can go on for years.'

She left. I could see that mentally she had crossed me off the list: I was a carer and so not in the running for any creative effort at this time. I supposed she was right but I felt discouraged. It was not that I was unused to God's 'lay-bys'. No missionary of twenty-eight years is worried about periods of waiting – waiting for permits, visas, job-descriptions, board decisions, planes that didn't fly. I was not arguing with God about this time of waiting. In fact, I saw it as very special 'training' for what I was about to do. But here I was, 'waiting' for my own father's death! The mixture of guilt and faith in the future was hard to handle.

'People don't die of dementia,' I was told more than once. 'And cancer grows very slowly in the old. It could be five or even ten more years.'

Good.
Or was it?

NOTE

1 Material from *Ageing*, A Report from the Board of
   Social Responsibility (Church House Publishing,
   1990) is copyright © The Central Board of Finance,
   and is reproduced by permission.

🎝 CHAPTER FOUR 🎝

Father was not in pain, or at least not in sharp pain. He was obviously uncomfortable sometimes, and we tried various types of pillows to help him sit with ease; but there were still things he enjoyed. Had he not suffered from dementia, I'm sure he would have lived these years contentedly.

What is it like to see your mind slipping away? I have heard people say to those who fear it for themselves (and who does not?), 'Never mind. At least you won't know if it happens to you.' But is this true?

The book *My Journey into Alzheimer's* is largely written by a man who, at the peak of his career as a Christian pastor, was told he had Alzheimer's – permanent, irreversible.[1] He knew what was happening for a long time, and maybe it was this fact that gave him periods of such darkness, when the peace and joy he had once enjoyed with the Lord disappeared and sleep brought a 'terrifying blackness'.

Perhaps in an older mind there is not such clarity of understanding about what is happening. Certainly father appeared to be at peace most of the day if we were around – at least if we weren't wanting him to do something! I wasn't so sure, however, about the nights.

Michael Ignatieff, who I only know as an occasional

writer in *The Observer*, talks about such people being 'prisoners of the realm of pure being'.[2] Butler and Orbach refer to it briefly in *Being Your Age*:[3]

> When, to all outward appearances, we are confronted with 'sans everything', it is not for us to judge that a person's selfhood has finally disappeared. What we contemplate is a mystery. All nature grows in the dark and it is God's providence which ordains who it is who needs that darkness of mind and sense in which the spirit can find its final consummation. We do not know at what perfection they are inwardly gazing, who endure this strange state of senile decay.

Perfection?

'He's so restless at night,' Gwen said to me, and I was aware of it as I sometimes sat with him or watched father sleeping. This is when I began to pray over him each night.

I became aware of evil spirits in Africa. We in the UK are slow to catch up on the African awareness of the spirit world. We are inclined to think of them as evil 'thoughts' – troubled dreams, a consciousness of an unease in a room or a house. Many of us experience them at night, especially at about 3 am!

Father often seemed troubled when he slept. Sometimes he would wake suddenly and ask a confused and anxious question about money or a house or other things that seemed to be on his mind.

'There's nothing to worry about,' Gwen would reassure him. 'Everything's fine.' But the reasoning mind was not there to drive such thoughts away.

I wondered. Could Satan see a wavering mind as a

chance to fill it with uneasy, doubting thoughts? Would God allow this? I didn't know the answer. All I saw was that his sleep was often troubled; so I 'stood at the gate of his mind' for him each night when he was asleep.

I first commanded any evil spirits present in the bedroom to leave in the name of Jesus. I spoke in a whisper, mainly because I didn't want to wake father, but also because I remembered reading somewhere that Satan cannot read our minds as God can and so we need to speak, however softly!

I used to say something like: 'I command you, evil spirits of fear and doubt, of lies and worry, of anger and frustration, to go from this room and this house in the Name of Jesus. Satan and all your minions, I raise against you the cross and the blood of Jesus and order you to leave. Go!'

Then I put my hand lightly on father and prayed, 'Holy Spirit of peace and love. Fill father's mind for him and give him peace tonight as he sleeps. Guard his mind from anxious thoughts and doubts. Fill it with your light and love.' I believe father slept more quietly after I started this.

One curious incident took place when I had been doing this for some time. I prayed as usual and remained in the dimly lit bedroom folding some clothes. Father suddenly seemed to wake up. He raised himself on his elbow and looked across at me. I saw he had recognised me clearly (itself unusual) and said, 'Did you get the victory?'

'Yes, I did,' I answered automatically.

Only afterwards did I wonder where that came from. Father had never used that kind of 'evangelical' language in my hearing. Nor had I ever used the phrase 'get the victory' in my nightly whispered prayers. What had been going on and what had he seen that made him ask this?

I feel that we, as Christians, have a special responsibility to those older brothers and sisters who are going through this particular valley of darkness. This is partly why I am a strong believer in the idea of Christian homes for those with Alzheimer's who cannot be cared for by relatives or friends. I will say more about this at the end of the book.

Another situation made me aware of the spiritual dimension of this disease.

Gwen and I often watched television in the evenings, and father would be sitting with us. It was a fairly easy time of the day. He could sit for hours just holding Gwen's hand as they used to in happier times, although he did not apparently take in much of what was happening on the screen. It was some time before I became conscious of how he was reacting to violent scenes.

Neither Gwen nor I particularly liked violent movies, but sometimes we were really too tired to notice or care much about which channel was on and occasionally we would look at a good thriller which inevitably had in it scenes of violence. I suddenly began to notice how father would wince at these scenes: the crashes, the blows, the cries, the police siren wailing as a criminal was cornered. Because of this, soon after I arrived in England, I bought a video recorder. It was the best investment I made.

Music always calmed father, and at that time Channel 4 ran something in the mornings called *The Art of Landscape* which was music while scenes of mountains and countryside were shown. Putting this on the video meant we could replay it later, when he was awake and alone in the bedroom, and it brought a lot of peace. Music from the proms, familiar scenes like the Trooping of the Colour or the Royal Tournament, films like *Mary Poppins* with light and colour and children, all were accepted peacefully. It made a big difference to him, not to be forced to see things that disturbed and irritated him because there seemed no sense in them.

I try not to think about the old people in hospitals and nursing homes forced to sit in front of a blaring set (because some are deaf) which is tuned to the 'most popular' channel. What happens to a mind that is already disturbed, when scenes of horror and violence are fed into it each day?

One other thing I remember concerning father's apparent 'awareness' of spiritual things. I have mentioned that his language had changed – he now used swear words much more than I ever remember him doing. Mild ones, admittedly, but they were still there.

We were used to him saying quite frequently, 'Oh God! Why can't you leave me alone?' But as time went on he suddenly started using the words 'Oh Christ!' quite a lot. I don't know why the latter worried me much more than the former. After all, basically they are the same. But it did. I winced every time I heard the name of my Saviour used like this.

In the end, one day when I was alone with him, I said, 'Dad, do you think you could stop using Christ as a swear word? It really does offend me very much.' This was at a time when he took in practically nothing of what we said and, if he did, did not retain it; but somehow that one got through. I never heard him say 'Oh Christ!' again. What channel to his mind was open to that request when so little of what anyone said was reaching him?

Sundays worried me. Sometimes the burden seemed heaviest on such a quiet day when no one called and even the street outside was empty of people. I wanted father to think of it as a special day – somehow. So I gave up going to the local church in the mornings and instead looked at the TV morning service with father, who was still in bed, just sitting by him and holding his hand. He would recognise hymn tunes sometimes and we would sing them together. How much he really took in I didn't know. Once, when an earnest young clergyman was preaching he said suddenly, 'Isn't it horrible?' Poor young man! So much for my efforts at 'keeping Sunday special'!

I went to church in the evening, when father was sitting by the fire in the sitting room and I felt Gwen could be left with him. The local Christians were sympathetic. They remembered father in happier times but, of course, few met him now.

'It must be very hard for you to see your father like this,' one lady said to me once.

'I don't think I really see him like this,' I answered. 'I see him either as he was, or as I think he will be when the Lord takes him.'

This was a genuine answer. I was not in any way repelled by what father had become; although if I unexpectedly came across earlier photos or memories of happier times – such as a 'diary' he kept for the family when we went on 'camping punt' holidays in the war! – it would hurt. But my daily mind saw him as I believe I will see him one day: in a new and shining resurrection body; and with a mind as God intended us to have – alert, alive, and joyful. This is something that we who spend much time with older people often forget: the resurrection body of the old, dribbling and muttering woman in the corner of the nursing home can and will, if she is a Christian, be as strong and as beautiful as any other in the life to come.

> Lo! I tell you a mystery. We shall not all sleep, but we shall all be changed, in a moment in the twinkling of an eye at the last trumpet. For the trumpet will sound, and the dead will be raised imperishable, and we shall be changed. For this perishable nature must put on the imperishable, and this mortal nature must put on immortality ... then shall come to pass the saying that is written, 'Death is swallowed up in victory.' *(1 Corinthians 15:51–54)*

Let us seek the lost among the old as earnestly and prayerfully as we do amongst the young. What if the passage there takes a hundred years, even more? Such periods are nothing compared with eternity.

Michael Ignatieff, in the article briefly referred to above,[2] wrote the following during the 1991 Alzheimer's Disease Awareness week:

> When we address one of the disease's central mysteries – why carers, by and large, remain so devoted to people the world calls vegetables – we need to stress something besides love and duty. We need to think of the disease as taking both carer and sufferer on a voyage together, which they know will leave them both utterly changed. It is a voyage of two people, inwards into the mind, into the realm of stillness.
>
> But only one of the travellers can return. Only

the carer will remember, only the carer will remain to pay tribute to their travelling companion, to the soul that has been left behind. This pact between the one who remembers and the one who can only forget is at the core of the relationship between care-giver and care-receiver. It is the pact that gives these relationships the strength to endure the fear and loathing on the way.

I have seen this pact give a person the strength to go the final distance into the dark. One traveller promises the other: I will be there at the end to see for the two of us. I will be there to tell them all what you once were like. I will remember. You will not be forgotten. Your suffering will not be senseless. The disease will not have defeated the two of us. One of us will return from the voyage to tell the tale.

Yes, I was travelling with father into a realm unfamiliar to us both – inwards into the mind – and trying to see something of what he saw there. It was changing him almost daily into someone different and yet, in essence, the same. It was changing me too as I went with him into the valley which I knew could only end in death.

What if there is no one who cares enough to go that final distance into the dark? What if the sufferer is alone? Then God is there who says:

Even to your old age I am He, and to grey hairs I will carry you. I have made, and I will bear. I will carry and will save.' *(Isaiah 46:4)*

We can only trust him, who created both mind and body, to hold them safe for us to reclaim most gloriously.

NOTES

1 *My Journey into Alzheimer's*, Robert Davis (Scripture Press, 1993).
2 © *The Observer*, 7 July 1991
3 *Being Your Age*, Michael Butler and Ann Orbach (SPCK, 1993), quoting from *On Growing Old*, S Harton (Hodder & Stoughton, 1957).

❧ CHAPTER FIVE ❧

Inevitably, life got more difficult. Broken nights became familiar as father would want to go to the loo several times and could no longer manage it on his own. Whether this was a genuine need or just something that his brain told him to do if and when he woke up, we were never sure; but it could be as many as four times through the night.

We collected, as time went on, an endless array of 'helping equipment': two varieties of a walking frame, bathroom accessories such as a high toilet seat, and many different bars and handles put in helpful places, but to get father to use them was a different matter. They were unfamiliar. He would rather put his hand on the insecure ironing board and the bookcase that had always been there. Early on, we were lent a commode wheelchair but, again, it was unfamiliar and we could not get father to sit in the chair, let alone use the commode.

As for walking sticks, no one had warned me of their ability to disappear completely the moment they were needed. If anything in this life 'merges' with the general furniture of a house more rapidly and effectively than a walking stick, I would like to know about it. We could have as many as two or three around the house, none of which were ever actually visible.

Gwen was entirely patient. I admired her greatly. She would get up at once, whether it was the first or the fourth time that night, help him to stand and then to walk the short distance to the bathroom. We had to be there. He could lose the way to the bathroom and turn towards the stairs, or mistake the bath for the toilet seat, try to sit on the edge and be in danger of falling backwards into it.

Helping a man who was over six foot to use the loo when we got there was also a struggle. Usually pants and pads needed to be changed. (Had we got them ready the night before?) Father would show bursts of anger.

'Get away!' he would say.

But we could not.

Anger was not difficult to deal with emotionally. Who wouldn't object to so much personal company in the bathroom? Sudden awareness of his situation was much worse. I remember once helping him change a pad when he was sitting on the loo. He looked down at the mess of blood and faeces.

'What is it?' he said pathetically, touching it with a finger.

'Nothing that matters, Dad,' I answered putting it into the bucket nearby and picking up a clean one.

He looked down at me kneeling at his feet doing for him what perhaps no daughter would expect to do for a father. Suddenly he was entirely rational and said gently, 'I'm so sorry, darling. So sorry.'

Those were the moments I knew what heart-break really was.

There were two of us – Gwen and myself. Could we have managed alone as most of those caring for Alzheimer's patients must surely do? Had I been alone in this situation, would I be writing about it now? Could I ever have 'come back to tell the tale'? I doubt it. There are some things better buried in the recesses of the mind and forgotten.

It was probably because we were two that we could fight the smells such a condition brings into a house. We were visited sometimes by my father's sister who had been a nurse all her life.

'How do you manage to avoid the smell?' she said. Auntie Kay was always practical!

In early months I sometimes would not wake for these nightly trips to the bathroom, but later on I had to because two were needed. Gwen would cope in the bathroom and I would deal with the bed that was often wet and needed changing, despite our care and use of plastic and rubber sheets. Before I had sometimes wondered how people coped with being constantly woken up at nights, like parents of young children or doctors on call; but now I realise it can, when needed, be built into one's lifestyle fairly easily. I learned to fall back into bed and go to sleep without much effort!

In the morning father was sleepy and it was, in some ways, the easiest time of day for us. I would bring him tea, which he rarely drank, and, much later, breakfast. He liked porridge, especially in the winter, which added to our bedclothes problem since no serviette or towel remained in place long. In the summer we went onto sugar puffs which were much easier to clear up. Gwen and I would have breakfast downstairs, mentally preparing for one of the more difficult times of the day which was getting him up.

Everyone had told us that he had to move. Lying in bed all day and all night could not be thought of: it would bring increased weakness, breathing difficulties and bedsores, something we in fact avoided throughout. But what a temptation it must be to some people – to leave such a person quietly lying there for most of the day. Again, I thought about other carers. Could they and would they, perhaps old themselves and tired out, struggle to get such a person up and washed every day? Wasn't it easier just to leave them. Even while writing this, I read in the national press of the difficulty of carrying out the statutory inspection system of private nursing homes. One inspector said, 'There was no doubt that some homes over-medicated patients to keep them quiet.'[1] I could understand, even if I could never condone.

'Time to get up, darling,' Gwen (or I) would say brightly.

'Oh hell!' was the answer. 'Can't you leave me alone?'

'Come on, Dad! It's nearly half past eleven.'

'Can't you go away?'

I suppose to him, comfortable now (having probably gone to the loo at about 4 am), it seemed cruel to be forced to get up. In fact, he even used that word occasionally: 'It's cruel! Why can't you leave me alone?'

We tried all sorts of ploys to persuade him – visions of coffee and the downstairs fire and 'Couldn't he help us by coming down because we wouldn't have to keep coming upstairs?' We sort of tugged at the duvet, only to have him pull back. Once (only once) I just pulled the covers right off the bed. That did the trick but I never did it again. It was the kind of thing you might do to a naughty child, and I felt ashamed.

Eventually, however, he would have to give in, and

the business of washing and dressing would begin. When he was downstairs – the stairs, well 'banistered' on either side, were never a real problem to him – and sitting by the dining-room fire with Gwen, a cup of coffee, and the morning paper on his knee, which he did not read but liked to have, he was happy. But the struggle to get him there was like a regular dentist's appointment every day.

The whole thing was hard work: fighting to keep the bathroom clean (by now we had plastic 'runners' on the floor), using the washing machine often twice a day, and pants all over the radiators (at least, before we realised our need of a tumble-drier). When ordinary things went wrong, they seemed much bigger than they were: a wasps' nest in the roof breaking through the ceiling just at the top of the stairs in the summer; pipes threatening to burst in the winter; drains blocking – the first (and, I hope, the last) time I had to discover just what happened and where when we flushed the loo. Ordinary household things seemed suddenly so hard to deal with.

But we were in a village and could find help. Mary came to clean twice a week; Joe came to cut the lawn from time to time, at least until the police discovered he had been growing cannabis in his garden. I went down the garden somewhat worriedly after that, eyeing perfectly innocent weeds suspiciously. The window cleaners came and went, even meals on wheels continued twice a week. Gwen and father had been getting these before I arrived and they continued. It was always good to see other people, and Fred, who brought the meals, was a shy but very courteous man.

'Good morning, sir!' he would say to father. 'How are you today?'

We so appreciated those who treated father as if he were a normal person. There is a tendency, when people get old, to treat them as children. One tries not to see it in homes.

'Come along, Maud dearie, bottoms up!'

'Oh dear! Din-dins on the floor again. Aren't we naughty?'

Perhaps they aren't all as bad as this, but the attitude is there.

Father sometimes went into the local hospital for a few days to give us a break. His name was Walter Hedley Taylor, but he had throughout his life been called 'Hedley'.

After one of these times, when he returned and I had to go and collect his 'washing' (which was usually a glorious collection of unknown clothing that we rather liked unpacking ... except that the pink pants were always there), one of the staff said to me, 'Walter doesn't answer to his name, does he?'

Sounded like a pet cat.

'Who doesn't?' I said, surprised. It hadn't occurred to me they wouldn't call him 'Mr Taylor'; but, understanding, I explained he was called Hedley.

'Oh, that explains it,' she said, satisfied.

Life went on: collecting the packets of pads from Swaffham hospital (a lifeline – how blissful to see the big cartons marked 'TAYLOR HIGHLY ABSORBENT'), putting them in black bags for the refuse collectors to take, and putting a few other things in with them so it wasn't so obvious what they were. Should they have been in 'red' bin bags anyway? What did people do with babies' disposable nappies?...

'Gwen! We've got a whole carton full of blue ones today!'

Of such were our pleasures. We did laugh sometimes and play silly games. I once wondered to Gwen
how often we went up and down stairs in the course
of the day. Since there was a convenient window-sill,
we put some red beans in one bowl and an empty
glass. Then, on Monday, every time I went up, I put
one bean in the glass and, on Tuesday she did the
same. I think it came out 25 against 24. Didn't sound
so much put like that.

But life 'outside' for both of us was almost at a
standstill.

NOTE

1 *The Guardian*, 26 August 1994, David Brindle,
   Social Services Correspondent.

CHAPTER SIX

'How long do you think your father is going to live?' people asked.

It was difficult not to wince, but I realised that some of them had the right to ask that before committing themselves to what I was doing.

In 1988, still employed in Kenya, I had sent out my first 'feeler' concerning the new ministry that I felt God was calling me to – that of reaching the old in the UK for Christ. It was a time of dreams and visions, which I referred to first in a small leaflet I sent out from Nairobi to different friends along with my ordinary prayer letter (with the kind permission of my missionary society). 'Where do dreams start?' I wrote then:

Perhaps in Africa: in the sun-drenched mountains of the highlands where space and distance and light brings peace to the heart; and the rising morning mist among the trees below lends itself to dreams. Or was it in the shade of the tall eucalyptus trees or deep-green mango trees, where the old sit, and talk washes gently back and forth: where the elderly are greeted kindly, respectfully? Where they matter.

Or did my dream also start in England, in the lines of closed doors and lonely people: in the cul-de-sacs of the housing estates and the small cottages of a country lane? How much of it was born from the sad and forgotten faces of the old as they shuffled through the Western supermarkets in a world of the young, the active, the money-spenders?

I suppose, humanly speaking, I owe much of my attitude to the old to twenty-eight years in Africa. I remember once giving a special meal to some Kenyan friends in Nairobi. There were some interesting Christian leaders among them, and I looked forward to the conversation since there were several issues dominating church life in Nairobi (and indeed, Africa) at the time. But I had made one mistake. One couple I invited were about fifteen years older than the others. This meant that whenever Joseph opened his mouth, the others fell silent to listen, and no one would contradict what he said. What 'elder' could resist that? On the whole, the party was not a success.

Of course, it was not always that kind of respect. Older 'country' people in Nairobi were tolerated rather than 'deferred to' in the cities.

'Hey, old man! The wild animals will eat you if you don't move faster than that!' called a lorry driver to an old country-dweller unfamiliar with crossing the road in a city. But it was kindly said. I compared it with a shout I heard in Swaffham when a motor cycle swerved to avoid a woman stepping off the curb: 'Get out of the way, you old bag!'

It bothered me to see how many older people were being treated this way in England, and to see the increasing fear of old age in so many.

When I was a new and young missionary living on

the high plateau of Ethiopia, which some call the 'roof of the world', I often used to spend a day visiting nearby villages. I would set out early, clutching my Amharic New Testament, with a Bible School student for company, sometimes climbing up through the hills for three or four miles to visit the distant villages that we could see far off, nestling in the rocks and little groups of trees.

Although we started early, the sun would soon grow hot and the dust from the feet of laden donkeys and mules sharing the narrow track with us would rise and blow in our faces. We would wind our way up the mountain slowly, and be so glad at last to arrive and sit on the mud 'benches' in the cool grass-roofed huts, drinking coffee, talking and teaching a little from flip-charts of pictures that the children loved. We would stay an hour or two, and then, as shadows began to lengthen, we would set out for home. Courtesy in Ethiopia demands that the host accompany a parting guest as far as the nearest stream, so all the family would come with us to the first rocky stream and wait while we crossed it.

'Go well!' the women would call out. 'Return in peace.'

I think I will never forget some of the glory of those walks home, along and down the hillsides in the waning sun: the colour of wild flowers, the spreading trees and darkening sky, the sight of cattle being slowly driven across the valleys into their compounds, and the calls of the herd boys. The dust lay on the path undisturbed, since the traders had long since passed and none would set out in the evening. The air was cool and fresh and the wind had dropped.

This scene often came back to me as a picture of

what our later years should be. We are tired as we grow old, for the strength of the morning has gone; but so has the heat and burden of the day. Our hearts are at peace: the day's task has been done – well or badly; it cannot be changed now for we are unable to re-live the past. The surging quest for recognition and significance in this competitive world has gone, and reflected in our eyes should be the distant glow which we know will get ever brighter – the glow of the opening gate.

What if we do have blisters? What if our backs are sore and we have bruised ourselves crossing a stream high up the mountain? What if memories of the mistakes we have made still haunt us? None of this matters. We are nearly home.

We watch others now – our children and grandchildren, if we have them, embark on journeys of their own – and we are glad; the mountains are still there to be explored. To see their strength, eagerness and youth will always be a joy, a reminder of our own morning climb. But we have no envy. We pass through this world but once, and we would not have it otherwise.

A quote attributed to Winston Churchill is recorded in a small book, *Thoughts on Life to Come*:[1]

> Let us treasure our joys – but not bewail our sorrows. The glory of light cannot exist without its shadows. Life is a whole, and good and ill must be accepted together. The journey has been enjoyable and well worth making ... once.

The memory of those evening walks in Ethiopia came back so often as this call to the elderly was growing more certain in my mind. This was surely the way to grow old: not with bitterness that life seems to be over, nor with anger at increasing disability and loss of faculties; but with the expectation of a future growing even brighter as we go on...

The path of the righteous is like the light of dawn, which shines brighter and brighter until full day. *(Proverbs 4:18)*

Perhaps I should not quote this without the assurance that heaven opens to us not because of our righteousness but because, through the cross, the righteousness of Christ can cover our forgiven sin: 'For our sake [God] made [Christ] to be sin who knew no sin, so that in him we might become the righteousness of God' (2 Corinthians 5:21).

What a comfort to us as we grow older and seem to look back on so much that needs forgiving. Once someone of another faith asked a Christian leader what word might encapsulate the special essence of the Christian faith. The answer was 'forgiveness'.

But what of those who have no faith, no expectation of anything except blankness and nothing? What of those behind the net curtains of a council flat, afraid to go out, with families far away from them? A survey taken a few years ago claimed that over one million old people in Britain did not have a visit from *one* person in seven days.

I wanted to go forward in evangelism. Nearly all my working life had been in the area of communication. Most of it had been teaching others how to communicate. 'Now, Lord,' I prayed, 'give me a chance to communicate, myself, the one great message that all others lead to: Christ and him crucified.' I longed to seek out older people, wherever they were, and tell them the good news of Christ; and I wanted to comfort and re-train(!) the depressed young curate who said to me once, 'It's really hard. There are only about six old people coming to the service.' I wanted to tell him, 'So what? They are still people, loved by God, capable of strength and beauty and life for eternity. Will the rejoicing in heaven be less because it is an old man of 70 coming to the Lord? Will the trumpets sound depressed, a little out of tune?

The 'only old'.

'I can't go to the Mothers Union/Women's Institute/ Ladies' Fellowship. There are only old people there.'

But not everyone was so pleased.

'Not *another* Christian organisation!' a friend groaned.

So I searched the *Christian Resources Handbook*: Youth for Christ, Youth with a Mission, Scripture Union... So much emphasis on young people. This was good, but who if anyone was targeting the old?

In 1989 I 'went public' and wrote an article for *Renewal* magazine called 'Growing Older'. In the article I asked, 'How is it that old age has become so feared, so ugly, so depressing a concept? What, in our society, has contributed to the isolation, the unwantedness of so many older people?'

At the end of the article was the information that I was 'interested in forming an evangelistic home mission in England aimed at reaching the over-60s for Christ'. I had over 80 responses (in fact, at 86 we stopped counting). So the vision had already, to some extent, 'taken off' before I even arrived in the UK. I was taken seriously and I was ready to go. I began to seek for prayer partners, both in Kenya and Britain, who would stand behind me in this new ministry.

When my move back to Britain finally did take place in June 1990, I had the full intention of starting 'Outlook' (by now it had a name) almost at once. But I was not the first of God's servants to find that there is often a period of waiting before a new ministry could begin. It was soon clear that the situation at home would take the major part of my time. From visiting people and telling them, 'I am starting a new ministry', I began to say, 'I am *hoping* to start...' And I cut down on such visits. It was unfair to take up the time of busy people when I was unable to move into the work I believed God was calling me to.

Some prayer partners (especially those who had been with me for some time) believed me, continued to pray for me and wrote encouragingly about 'the Lord's perfect timing'. Other contacts simply lost interest. Small gifts of money continued to come, which enabled my bedroom/office to exist: a desk, a small computer, even a filing cabinet were bought in this period; but I recognised that it was difficult for people who knew nothing about me to take my visions seriously at this stage.

I visited my local bishop who was largely uninterested. 'Come back to me when it's more than a gleam in your eye,' he said.

I tried not to blame him.

There was a time in my life when I was involved in the formation of what has become a large Christian University in Nairobi. I was one of the team who wrote up the first published catalogue, so learning in the process how to write 'course descriptions'. There were over a hundred of them.

In a letter to my African prayer partners during this period I wrote, half-humorously, a course description for what I called an 'independent study' with God – 'Care of the Old (Field study)':

A period of close involvement with the aged in need of special care. The course will involve caring for those suffering from Alzheimer's (dementia), terminal cancer, and other age-related illnesses as well as contact and discussion with those caring for such people on a regular basis. Residential homes, wards for the elderly in hospital, and psychiatric units will be visited and some practical work undertaken. Related reading will bring to the participant some understanding of the situation of the elderly who are in need in Britain today.

I believed that, when I had enough 'credits' in God's training school, he would move me on. But it wasn't always easy.

NOTE

1   Extract from *Thoughts on Life to Come*, Mary Oakley (Tim Tiley Prints, Bristol, 1981, revised 1993).

CHAPTER SEVEN

My father sits the other side of the fireplace, looking as he ever did. He seems to long to talk.

'Are we going to go?' he says.

'Where to?' I ask gently. 'Is there somewhere you would like to go?'

'Yes, I'd like to … well … you know … to … well, I wanted to … Oh, never mind!' The programme could not finish.

'Going' anywhere was a real problem. The time came when the 'respite care' given in the local hospital could not continue. There were staircases around, and the service provided was not set up for those with dementia. On the other hand, we had to have some break from the increasing strains of 24-hour care. We were fortunate in that there was a special unit in Kings Lynn (about twenty miles away) that was willing to take him in. Initially, we were given one week in six.

Gwen and I paid it our first visit. Certainly the newly built unit was good, the rooms spacious and clean. We were prepared, at least partly, to accept that there would be many people like father there. Even so, the sight of an old man ambling down the wide corridor with a long string of mucus coming from his nose was unnerving, especially when he tried so hard to open the (coded) door that we had just come through. One of the staff saw our distress.

'Come along, George,' she said kindly to the man. 'Nearly time for tea', and led him away.

One of the big advantages of the place was that it was spacious with many open doors, so those who felt they had to be on the move could wander around safely. There was even a French window leading out into the walled garden.

A woman dressed for the street passed us, heading for the window. She put her finger to her lips,

'Shh!' she said. 'Don't tell anyone. I'm going out.'

I thought she was a staff member until I saw her wandering aimlessly around the walls, looking for the door which was not there.

The 'day room' had in it the usual number of arm-chairs and tables. ITV was on the television (although not loudly), coloured magazines on the table, some flowers – and some people who seemed to our nervous gaze to be the wrecks of human existence. But there was kindness also.

An old lady in a pink dressing gown was coming down the corridor looking lost. She saw me and I smiled. She held out her hand, like a child waiting to be led. I took her into the day room and sat beside her holding her hand while she smiled at me and was calm.

How touch mattered to father. What calmed him more than any other thing was the touch of a human hand. He would reach for Gwen's hand so often – or mine – and be content to hold it in his for hours.

What is it about human contact? What passes between one human being and another when we touch? Why did touching us calm father? I am sure feelings travel through such contact. If we were distressed and upset, he would somehow feel it too and become restless and unhappy. 'Are you all right?' he would ask continually. 'Are you all right?' Equally, as I claimed the peace of God and held his hand, at peace myself, he would be calm and smile at me.

I dreaded the thought of his coming into this institution, good though it was. Who would care how distressed he appeared here? Who would answer him when he asked for Gwen? What would happen when he struggled to resist washing or getting up? Would he feel lost without those he was used to around him?

It was useless to torment myself with such thoughts. It had to happen. We had not the strength to continue without a break.

'It'll be good for him to have a change,' my brother assured me down the phone. 'It will stimulate his mind.'

On that first visit – made without father (we must have been sent a carer) – Gwen made arrangements with the staff of the home; we said our goodbyes and successfully managed the code on the door to get out. Once out of that department, Gwen and I walked down the quiet corridors trying to pretend we had not been horrified by the sight of so many sufferers from dementia put together. We lost our way. The corridors were long and there were so many of them.

Suddenly a burst of maniacal laughter echoed from a nearby room. We gripped each other, paling physically. What kind of 'dement' laughed like that? Then I saw a glass panel in a nearby door and looked through it.

'It's all right,' I said through dry lips to Gwen. 'It's only the cleaners!'

A number of women in blue overalls were obviously having a coffee break.

On the day father was to go, we needed to get him up and dressed so that he would be ready for the ambulance that was coming to fetch him. This was a struggle since it was earlier than usual. Then we were informed that the ambulance had been called to a road traffic accident and could not come. Would we bring him ourselves, or wait until the next day? It was like the last day of the school term when I was a teacher. One felt one could not last one more day! Father was dressed and ready, despite the struggle it had been to get him so; his bag was packed. The prospect of delay was intolerable. We decided to take him ourselves in the car.

One of our helpers was there at the time, or we would never have managed to persuade him to step outside the front door into the waiting car. He struggled and fought. I bit my lip until it nearly bled.

'Come on, Dad. It's only going to the doctor. You know you go to the doctor sometimes.'

We did not try to put on the seat-belt – it would have been too difficult. He sat in the front next to me, and I drove to Kings Lynn with Gwen in the back.

After father started respite care, he hardly ever recognised 'home' again. He was deeply distressed: 'Where are we going? It's horrible. When are we going home?'

When we got there, we could not get him out of the car. The staff came with a wheelchair, and we tried to coax him out of the front seat.

'Come along, Mr Taylor. There's a nice cup of tea inside.'

Gwen tried to persuade him, 'I'm coming in too, darling. Just for a little while.'

'Get the hell away from me! Leave me alone!'

I joined in, 'Come on, Dad. The doctor's waiting to see you. You know you always go to the doctor.'

He looked at me with that sudden clear comprehension I had come to dread. 'If I get out, you'll drive away and leave me here,' he said.

That was the end of my participation in the event. I left them all abruptly and disappeared into the hospital grounds. Gwen was left to help them finally persuade him out and wheel him into the hospital. She went in to stay and have a cup of tea with him. It was a cold day, and twice staff came to find me and ask me to come in and join them. But I could not. The car, parked in front of the main entrance, stayed there until Gwen came out, and I drove her home trying to forget the fear of being left that I saw in my father's eyes. I hope that when I am in my nineties I will be loved enough for such tears to be shed for me.

Father went a number of times to the 'respite care' unit in Kings Lynn. It was always difficult to get him there, although it was easier if he went by ambulance – the men would cheerfully get him into a wheelchair and carry him downstairs before he knew what was happening to him. It was true (as my brother had said) that he was slightly more alert each time he came back, and would be inclined to do more for himself – perhaps begin to get dressed or comb his hair on his own. But he was also more confused and sometimes didn't even recognise us or his home. Once, on the first night home, we were disturbed every two hours with his getting up for no reason that we knew of. We 'went to the loo' because it was what he did in the night: not because he needed to. (What had happened in the care unit?)

Once, during a 'respite care' week, Gwen and I were called by the doctor in charge for an 'assessment meeting'. Father was brought in and sat in a chair. There were about ten people in the room. I never knew who they all were but suspected several of them were students or trainee nurses. There was a social worker I knew, and a member of staff that Gwen and I used to call privately 'Irma Greaser' (after the woman who made lampshades out of human skin during the war). I should add that on the whole the staff were kind and helpful. I can't remember what this poor woman had done in front of us to earn that nickname!

Although the doctor was competent and helpful, the meeting was difficult to say the least. This was because it was so 'public' and because father was there, waving his head about in confusion – an object presumably of medical interest. (Were they making notes about him?) It was my first experience of what many must know about in similar situations, when you cease to be an individual and become 'the wife' or 'the daughter'. I gripped the arms of my chair and saw the notebooks flutter. I imagined the entry: 'Daughter appears tense and hostile...'

Next time it happened, we asked for fewer people to be present and also that father not be asked to 'attend'. But the respite care we were offered kept us going. We were immensely grateful for it.

❦ CHAPTER EIGHT ❦

Sometimes I kept a diary…

7 December 1991

We have started leaving father upstairs in bed most of
the morning. It is such a struggle to get him up and
down stairs that we have decided to give him breakfast in bed and then get him up for lunch. But I worry
sometimes that he lies up there for so long. The bedroom is large and chilly, although he is always warm
in bed. But what is he thinking about as he lies for
hours semi-awake at that time of day, as the winter
sun streams through the window?

He always seems glad to see me when I go in. 'Is it
there?' he will ask anxiously, although we never know
what he means by that. Perhaps it is the result of his
latest dream. I know he does have troubled dreams
sometimes. Gwen tells me he will awake in the night
and talk confusedly about paying bills or getting
money from a bank. She reassures him, 'Don't worry
about it. We have enough money.'

For me, it is the first time for nearly thirty years that
I have experienced an English winter from start to finish. Most missionaries from warmer countries make
sure that they don't. If my 'missionary leave' was due
in the winter, I used to make sure that I stayed for

Christmas and the New Year and then went back to the sun some time in January, just when it was getting really cold with snow on the horizon.

Now I stand in the bedroom and look out in dismay at the sodden and colourless garden. Suddenly, the shabby chicken huts through the back-wire and the old tin barrel we once used as an incinerator are in view through the bank of dead nettles. Even – could it be? – signs of an old and sodden deck-chair cushion under the bushes near the fence. I wish we'd had the lawn cut once more before all this started.

We take him breakfast in bits – sugar puffs and cut-up apple. I would like to take him porridge on these cold days and we do sometimes, but eating porridge in bed does unspeakable things with the bedding and everything else around.

The main difficulty is that he lies on the right-hand side of a double bed and so leans over to eat with his left hand. To sit up with a tray is something we cannot get him to do. Any change (such as to change the bed or his place in it) is really not worth the struggle to achieve. Familiarity gives reassurance and quietness, and that is far more important.

Coffee and toast and marmalade are a little easier. 'Thank you, darling. That's lovely,' he says.

10 December 1991
I have taken a small lighted Christmas tree upstairs. It brightens the room which, by 3.30 pm, is almost dark. Father lies and watches it.

'It's a Christmas tree,' I say and he says, 'Yes. Isn't it pretty?'

We would do anything to make his life a little more worth the living.

12 December 1991

I think pain must be beginning now. When he wants to go to the loo, you can see him shifting in his chair downstairs, even though we have used all kind of cushions to ease him. He is out of bed now for five or six hours a day but, despite the struggle it is to get him upstairs again, he is always glad to get back.

People are kind. A lady at the church gave me a mohair scarf for his shoulders in bed yesterday. Rather to my surprise he likes it as we tuck it around him. She had said, 'I'll have it back sometime' and I smiled to myself. Usually things he uses aren't in a fit state to be 'given back'. Already I've had to scoop porridge and pieces of marmaladed toast out of it.

His pyjamas are a problem. They need renewed elastic and various buttons. Neither Gwen nor I have talents in that direction although I can (and do) sew on buttons. What is one supposed to do about stretched elastic on otherwise sound pyjama bottoms? It's easier to get a few more pairs at Swaffham market.

15 December 1991

We had a visitor yesterday evening – an older lady who used to live next door and was very fond of father. She had moved to Swaffham, and I had to go and fetch her in a quite-frightening fog. I am not used to winter driving in England. The way the fog sometimes 'hangs' over the road in a kind of very low cloud is unnerving, and I haven't found the knack of locating the right turn to the village when I can't see anything but the muddy nearside verge.

Father sits quietly when someone else is there – glad, I think, not to have the burden of making sure that we are 'all right'. This is a phrase he must use twenty times a day if we are not actually conversing. 'Are you all right?' he will ask if we are perhaps watching a TV programme or reading the newspaper.

'Yes, darling. We're fine.'

Fifteen minutes later: 'Are you all right?'

'Yes. We're fine.'

When a visitor is there whom he feels comfortable with, he smiles and looks from one to another as we talk. No one watching would think there was anything wrong.

He likes the evenings, especially if both Gwen and I sit with him in the sitting room. He obviously feels safe and happy there, and sits in his usual chair holding Gwen's hand. But 'anchoring' us means a lot of work later on as we wash up, take the washing out (and the pipes have frozen in the outhouse so at the moment we can't do any), make the bed, set out his pants (in which we pin the pads) and so on.

This pants business is really something. You're meant to keep the incontinence pads on with what looks like net underpants. But they were not intended for a man over six foot who is hostile at once to anything unfamiliar. When we tried them he would pull the pads out with irritation. 'What are these things?'. We have found the only solution is to use safety pins and pin the pads into the clean underpants so they looked just like ordinary pants. We do this six or seven times a day, trying to keep up. We have become experts on safety pins: so has the washing machine.

Our friend, elderly herself, was kind and understanding, accepting him as he was without much comment. He does, after all, look physically very well indeed. She made Gwen smile by reminding us how, when she visited us, father would slip out to the shop across the road and come back with ten cigarettes for her.

16 December 1991

I have found out what to do about finding a right turn in a fog. Old Mr Matthews told me in the shop. He says you drive on to the next left turn (which will tell you where you are) and then turn around so that the right turn you want is a left turn. I must try it.

18 December 1991

I took the day off yesterday to visit London: just to shop a little, see the Christmas lights, and go to a theatre with a friend. We went to *The Lion, the Witch and the Wardrobe*. It was a matinee and full of school children. We sat in the back row of the stalls and pretended we were headmistresses.

Gwen was upset and irritable when I returned early next morning. I know it is because she no longer feels she can cope alone with father.

'I had a dreadful day yesterday. I don't know how long I can go on,' she says. I felt resentment rise in me that I could not leave the house even for twenty-four hours without being made to feel guilty.

Gwen's fear had communicated itself to father who also was bad-tempered and angry.

'Oh Christ! Why can't you leave me alone!' he said as I tried to give him breakfast and, pushing me away, he upset the coffee on the clean sheets. The whole atmosphere in the house was hostile and fearful. Was it because for a day and a night no prayer had been uttered there? Was Satan that near, seeking entrance?

I began to pray inwardly at once, commanding Satan and his evil servants of fear and anger to leave the house in the all-powerful name of Jesus. How I love that name: Jesus. Jesus. I felt father begin to calm down and a sense of quiet also began to return to me. I dare not cease to call: Jesus! Jesus! He was there, 'fulfilling the desire of them that fear him' (Psalm 145:19). The day will begin to change now…

26 December 1991
What a Christmas! For the first time in my life, I am glad it is over.

Whether because father was conscious of 'different things' (like the tree and the lights and the cards downstairs or the unfamiliar quietness on the street outside) or whether we were getting tired even by the modest kind of preparation we were involved in, I don't know. But he did seem to become more difficult and uneasy. It took us longer to persuade him to do anything at all, and he spilt more and generally opposed all our suggestions.

On Christmas Eve, Gwen went to have her hair done. This was a weekly event and important. I recognised the need to keep up normal activities as much as possible, and make an effort at our own appearance. She usually drove herself into the local town for it. But today she was tired and upset, and the town would be like a market day only worse. Parking would be impossible. I decided I should run her in, leave her, and she could get a taxi back. Father had finished his breakfast and was usually quiet at this time of day.

The trip took me twelve minutes. When I got back, father had got up, been to the bathroom (and missed the loo entirely), returned, sat, still wet on his bed, winding the mohair scarf around his hips. He was shivering and confused. It took at least an hour to straighten things out.

I don't (even inside, thank God) get angry at father at these times. (How I would react in any Nursing Home at anyone who did, I don't know...) I sat down beside him and coaxed him into getting dressed, padded-up, and sitting in the chair by the bed. Then we had a cup of coffee and I turned the television on.

I then removed the duvet cover, adding it to the washing, took the first lot to the washing machine, and started on the really soiled stuff in the bath. Let no one think (if they do) that you can pick up faeces-covered sheets or underwear and put them straight in the machine. A pre-wash is needed. I then lifted the plastic floor covering to scrub it and started hand-washing the mohair scarf.

Kneeling over the bath, working on some of the worst, I looked around for Satan and addressed him.

'You think this is a great Christmas Eve for me, don't you? Well, let me tell you I am still praising the Lord for the gift of his Son. This is his house, his day, and I am rejoicing in him!'

That shut him up for the moment.

If anything, Christmas day was probably worse. Father suddenly cannot seem to keep urine under any control. Up to now it has mainly been faeces. We were both up four times in the night and at least twice had to entirely change the bed linen despite the plastic sheets. At least the mattress was still protected. Sensing the difference, father was more troubled.

'It's coming down,' he kept saying.

By eight in the morning, father was still going to the loo every half hour or so because, I think, he now felt himself wet and the feeling was unfamiliar. Gwen couldn't take any more and I took over, dressing him in grey track-suit trousers. I went to fetch something from downstairs and, when I returned, he was wandering around clutching his groin. It was soaking wet. Help! Gwen was 'beat' and doing vegetables in the kitchen. I got him back to the loo (which, of course, he didn't now need) and sat him there while I searched for more clothes and pads. I tried, clumsily and unsuccessfully, to pin two pads together: eight pints doesn't seem so much now. Finally, we got him downstairs where he stayed for some hours,

We had a good lunch but, as a day, it was not a success! Father seemed more and more confused and upset. He talked a lot – mostly nonsense, which worries Gwen, who tries to make sense of it, more than me who just follows it along. But even *my* mind began to reel as the day wore on.

In the middle of the day I went off with a friend to do meals on wheels in the villages around. Some of our regulars had been taken away by relatives. Those who remained were not in celebratory mood.

An old couple in a lonely, isolated cottage: neither could move without pain, the fire was scarcely burning, and the husband was pale and sallow with a flu bug.

A blind lady who was not normally on our list; she was in bed. 'It's too cold to get up. Who are you? What do you want? Where do you come from?'

A bad-tempered man in a village at least six miles away, and his brother. He had ordered two meals and the brother was making the best of it.

Old Mrs White was still insisting on being served through the front window – it was too painful to reach the door.

Happy Christmas, everyone. Where is it?

Well, maybe spending it like this reminds us of the reality in that stable in Bethlehem. Who washed the cloths out after the delivery? Who cut the cord and removed the afterbirth? Who if anyone washed the baby and with what sort of water? Was there a loo? (Was it outside? I bet it smelt.) Was there enough light, and did the lantern smell of rancid oil? How much animal dirt was there? And did they really want strangers pushing their way in just when they had begun to relax a little?

Christmas. We have covered it with tinsel and pretty wrapping-paper. But underneath the suffering goes on. Which is the real Christmas?

❧ CHAPTER NINE ❧

The winter went on and on. Whereas in Nairobi or Addis Ababa the world was always light, active and moving by 6.30 to 7 am, now at 8 or 8.30 the Norfolk village was totally dark and silent. I used to wake (from habit) between 6 and 6.30 and wonder where the world had gone. At breakfast I would stare, hungry for light, out of the window. Was this the best it was going to do?

But it was good to be part of a family, even in these circumstances. In Africa it was assumed by some Africans that a single Western missionary just didn't have a family or, if they did, that it really wasn't that important to them.

'I have to go home this weekend,' the church Provincial Secretary, a Kenyan of my own age, used to tell me. 'My brother is in real trouble.' Then he would add with a rather smug smile, 'You know, to us, the family really matters.'

It matters to me too, I used to think. Giving up close links with my family in England, being unable to get to know and love nephews and nieces, brothers and sisters, was one of those 'missionary sacrifices' I was trained to make in the 60s, before 'short-term service' came in and all the nephews and nieces started driving mini-buses around Africa. But I recognised that everyone, if they could, is created to be in some kind of family and, much as I loved the African families who took me on board, I missed my own.

So to be seen by the village as 'Mr Taylor's daughter come home from Africa to look after him' was not a bad thing. It gave me an identity, a place in the community. But it played havoc with the inside 'me', a servant of God called into a new ministry. Time just disappeared in cooking, shopping, cleaning, filling forms, paying bills – ordinary household things that I wasn't very good at. Months rushed by. 'The future' was temporarily on hold. I fought not to let the present swallow me up entirely and I became spiritually very thin and hungry.

I copied out in my diary:

> If I neglect communion with God and don't make knowing and hearing his voice a top priority, how will I escape Satan's deception in these trying days? ... [It will be a] dangerous, deadly neglect. A weakened deteriorating spirit. Deception. Destruction ...[1]

But how did one keep 'spiritually fit' in this kind of situation? Where were the quick-thinking, challenging companions of the African media world? The Bible studies? The church services with hundreds present? Was I supposed to be satisfied with a twenty-minute sermon once a week in a village church with a congregation of 20 plus, and a set of Scripture Union Bible study notes? And where was the *sun* in this cold land?

Humanly speaking, the tape-ministry saved me. I used the Anchor Recording Bible Study tapes obtainable on hire, and I borrowed out-of-date but still good books from the church library. Some I had read before, such as *Against the Tide* by Watchman Nee.[2]

> The will of God may be clear and unmistakable, but
> for us His way to it may sometimes be indirect. Our
> self-esteem is fed and nourished because we say 'I
> am doing the will of God!' and it leads us to think
> that nothing on earth should stand in the way of
> that. Then one day God allows something to fall
> across our path in order to counter that attitude…
> …We do not accomplish God's work merely
> by yielding to the appeal of open doors and great
> opportunities. There is also very often a dark night
> to be endured with patience for the sake of a new
> life…'

The struggles of those early missionaries in China
continued to speak to me:

> …the timing was profoundly reassuring…. If they
> would press on humbly, keeping close to God, the
> care of all the consequences was surely His.

The timing. What was the timing?

A year and a half passed. I was 58. 'Be ready for five
or six years, even ten, Rhena,' the medical visitors
warned kindly. But I could never see it like that. God
did not play with us. This would end at the right time.

'When do you think your father will die?' I was
often asked this: by friends interested in the new pro-
ject; by my step-brother, concerned about the strain on
his mother; by villagers who wanted to have an idea
of how ill father really was; by African friends writing
or phoning to see how I was.

I did not know, but I knew it would be in God's perfect time.

I studied hyacinth bulbs growing. Once, by accident, I knocked one of the flower-pots over when the shoot was about an inch high and I had just removed it from the dark cupboard it had started life in. Collecting the compost and bulb to replace them in the pot, I was astonished at the number of roots the bulb had grown. They almost filled the pot. 'All nature grows in the dark.' Where had I heard that?

Well, I was going to grow in the dark!

The (then) BCMS[3] paid me for six months after my return. They had supported me for thirty-one years and I had no complaints. It was strange, certainly, not to 'belong' anywhere in the Christian sense. I found having to end relationships with BCMS 'partner churches' unexpectedly hard, rather like being sent away from a foster home. One minute you seem to belong and be relatively important to them. The next they have 'adopted' somebody else, and the missionary board at the back of the church is all about 'Shirley Packard' or 'Graham McAllister' instead of you.

A shrinking world.

I was quite ignorant of the 'benefit' system in the UK. One of our advisors had helped Gwen get the attendance allowance for father. Much later, a nice young man in the job centre suggested I apply for invalidity benefit. I queued up with everyone else on Saturday mornings and received £31.25 a week. So far so good.

I didn't know much about doctors either. Once, early on, when Gwen was visiting her family and I had been left alone with father for several days, I asked someone to stay with Dad and went to see his doctor whom I had not met before.

'He seems so distressed at night,' I said. 'I can't get him up to bed and when he's in bed he always wants to get up. I was wondering about some kind of sleeping pill.'

He was sympathetic but unwilling to prescribe sleeping pills. 'You never know the effect of them on someone like your father,' he said.

Just as I was leaving, he said, 'Are you alone? You do know people in that condition can turn violent, don't you?'

'I've heard it,' I said, and left.

Neither Gwen nor I could ever imagine father harming either of us. Dr L was probably a reasonable GP. I know Gwen had found him so with earlier problems she had with father, when cancer was first diagnosed. It's just that I didn't know much about doctors.

He did call from time to time. If Gwen was there, he would greet her cheerfully and go and see father, who greeted him as politely as any other visitor who wasn't asking him to do anything.

'Well, how are you?' the doctor would say breezily.

'Oh, I'm fine,' Dad would answer.

He would take his pulse but I never saw him do anything else.

Once or twice I was alone when the doctor came, and occasionally he seemed to want to talk over coffee or a glass of sherry. He once enlarged on his great number of elderly patients.

'We put them in homes just when their life is drawing to a natural end,' he said, 'and then they just stop struggling and thinking for themselves and go on living because there's nothing else to do.'

'Do you think they want to?' I asked.

'Go on living? Probably not. But once they're in a home and their needs are being met, they just can't die.'

It was one way of looking at things.

On another occasion he came when I was really tired.

'How long are you going to stay?' he asked me abruptly.

'I suppose as long as I'm needed,' I answered. 'Gwen can't manage alone.'

He nodded. 'Well, remember you can simply walk away from it all,' he said. 'So can your step-mother, come to that. Then the State has to take over.'

'Just walk away.' I remembered this but still think it poor comfort. I loved my father and could not 'walk away'. Not yet, anyway.

NOTES

1 *The Hearing Ear*, Larry Lea (Harvestime Publishing Limited, 1988).
2 *Watchman Nee – Against the Tide*, Angus Kinnear. Published by Kingsway Publications copyright © 1973 Angus I Kinnear.
3 Bible Churchman's Missionary Society, now re-named CROSSLINKS.

❧ CHAPTER TEN ❧

In the dreariest month of the year, when the winter was at last showing a faint sign of ending and a few grimy aconites were showing above the soil, my aunt died – my father's sister. She was 91, two years younger than my father. She had been the only girl in a family of boys. Their parents had been missionaries for CIM (Church Inland Mission) in China, and I have an early 'prayer card' of my grandparents, dated 7 October 1901, when Kay had been a babe in arms and my father a toddler just able to stand.

'Auntie Kay' had always been a practical and essential part of our family circle. Unmarried, a nurse and later a 'health visitor', she had been always on hand for the various crises which most families go through. Just prior to my return from Kenya to look after my father, she had left Maidenhead and moved unexpectedly to a Norfolk Abbeyfield Home. I had been surprised at the time for, although father and I and another branch of the family were in Norfolk, her friends were all in Maidenhead.

'I want it to be easy for you all to come to my funeral,' she said when I asked her why she had moved.

'But you're not about to die,' I said, for she had good health and still seemed well.

She did not answer.

But we liked her being in Norfolk. Sometimes when a 'sitter-in' came, Gwen and I used to go to the Fakenham Abbeyfield (about half an hour's drive away) and eat our lunch sandwiches in her room. She was always understanding and encouraging about our situation, sympathising, advising where she could.

Then she fell ill and I went to her in Fakenham.

'I think I might be going to pip your father at the post,' she said, trying to smile.

I drove home through the tunnels of leafless trees, and remembered how she used to talk to me about death.

'I don't mind death, Rhena,' she used to say. 'It's just *how* I die.'

She told me about a friend of hers who had lived alone and died at night on her way to the loo. The police had broken in when Kay had reported the curtains were still drawn one morning.

'They tried to stop me going in,' Kay said. 'But I saw Jessie … all uncovered. It was so undignified, and she had been so modest and careful about her body.'

The thought had preyed on her mind.

I tried to comfort her. 'It was only her body. People understand.'

What sort of death would hers be? Would father's be?

Her sickness at this time was one other awful thing to happen, when Gwen and I felt we had all we could manage. Kay was taken to a Norwich hospital and I needed to visit her. But father could not be left for long, and Gwen now found it very difficult to be left alone with him. I was divided between being at home and spending time at the hospital in Norwich which was thirty-six miles away. I seemed to be moving in a kind of nightmare.

Kay had a lump to the side of her body. Her bowel was affected and she was in pain.

'They're going to find out what it is,' she told me.

'It could be some kind of obstruction, couldn't it?' I said hopefully. 'Has it just come?'

'No. It's been there for over two years.'

'And you've never said anything?'

'I didn't want that operation ... I've seen too many of them.'

'What operation?'

'Removal of the bowel. Bags to empty. Smells.'

I was silent but I thought about that as I drove home. Kay was a nurse and she must have had a good idea of what the lump growing inside her was likely to be. She had made the decision to be silent and die from it. She didn't want to struggle on with all the difficulties an operation would have led her to. How many others would have the courage to make such a decision? Was it a right one to make? Had I known, had other members of the family known, would we have insisted she told her doctor so that something could have been done? I don't know and probably, because she knew how difficult it would have been for us, Kay never told us or shared that decision with us. How many other old people choose their time to die?

Father had been having heart problems before I came home. I never knew exactly what these were but it was enough for him to have to take pills regularly. I remember them because, on earlier home leaves from Africa, I heard him joke about the 'red, white and blue' pills he was supposed to take at different times during the day. Once dementia had him in its grip, no one ever mentioned the pills again. The implication hovered – if his quality of life was so low, let us not seek to prolong it.

My visits to Kay were short. Gwen needed me at home. Kay and I used to pray a little together at the hospital. She was a Christian, if not a very vocal one.

She hated dependency. Once she was nearly crying because a young orderly had been impatient and unpleasant at having to take her to the loo. We tried to help her. The other family branch, living much nearer Norwich, took the brunt of the visiting.

'I have to have another operation,' she said after a week had passed.

Amazingly, just at that time, there was a conference in the conference centre in the village where we lived, and a third call was made on my time. Christian leaders were gathered there whom I knew and would, in normal times, have been glad to talk to. I made brief appearances.

'I'm fine, thank you,' I would say. 'It's great to be in England. God will show me when to start the work he has called me into. What's happening to you?'

The weather remained dank and miserable. Kay grew weaker. Car parking at the hospital was consistently difficult. In her pain, near death, Kay remained aware of my situation.

'You mustn't stay,' she used to say feebly. 'Gwen needs you at home.'

We were not with her twenty-four hours a day.

I asked the ward sister, 'What happens if she dies and no one is with her?'

She answered simply, 'If we see death is really near, several of us will stay with her.'

I arrived soon after the second operation. I had to park in a multi-storey some distance from the hospital. She was on a trolley about to be taken back into the operating theatre.

'Where are you going?' I asked her. 'I thought it was over.'

'I need to be taken back,' she said, and I saw the consciousness that she was dying in her eyes. I had not been so close to the 'valley of the shadow' before.

'Remember you're safe in his arms,' I whispered. 'There's nothing to worry about.'

She nodded. 'I've pipped your father at the post, haven't I?' she said weakly smiling as some orderlies came for the trolley.

I hesitated, wondering what to do. She saw it.

'Go home,' she said, and I could only just hear her. 'You're needed.'

She died before they could operate again.

We did not try to tell father.

I remembered an African song I had heard at many funerals in Africa, in which the one who has died is seen to be on a moving train going towards heaven; those of us left behind stand watching and waving on the platform. The song, using a strong 'train-rhythm beat', calls a goodbye after those on the train and sends messages to those who had already gone ahead to heaven. Messages are even sent to Moses and Paul and Elijah! What a sense of the reality of heaven was in their hearts.

I too gained something by being with Kay as she drew near to the Kingdom. I almost felt myself straining to see with her who waited for her on the other side of the river.

Now we know that if the earthly tent we live in is destroyed, we have a building from God, an eternal house in heaven, not built by human hands ... For while we are in this tent, we groan and are burdened, because we do not wish to be unclothed but to be clothed with our heavenly dwelling, so that what is mortal may be swallowed up by life. *(2 Corinthians 5:1,4)*

Kay's funeral was quiet. Gwen and I went to the short service at the crematorium near Norwich. We had managed to get a 'carer' but she only had two hours to spare. We were, perhaps, twenty in number at the funeral – to mark the ending of a life spanning nearly a century and several continents.

African funerals bring hundreds together for, sometimes, days of mourning and feasting. Families are often impoverished by the food bill and the cost of bringing all the many relatives from different parts of the country. Here in the West it seems funerals scarcely ripple the surface of life and are just a quiet goodbye from those who love the one dying, and who also happen to be near at the end. Since Kay had deliberately chosen to leave the place where she had lived most of her life to be near us, she had her wish. It was too difficult for many from Maidenhead to come but it was 'easy' for us, as she had wanted.

The young clergyman knew none of us. 'We come together to mark the passing of this old lady,' he said.

Everyone of us stiffened. Whatever Kay had been, she had not been 'an old lady'!

I used to be surprised at how quickly people in general got used to a death. The circle closes so quickly, as if we are afraid to leave a gap there too long. I discovered with Kay's death that the circle might close, but the gap stays in the hearts of those who close it. Gwen and I both missed her very much.

❧ CHAPTER ELEVEN ❧

'Where's Gwen?' father asked, catching my hand as I passed his chair.

It was a question I had heard a hundred times before. The only difference now was that Gwen was actually in the room.

'I'm here, darling,' she would say.

'Oh … yes. But what is this room?'

'It's your sitting room, in your own house.'

'But where's Gwen?'

'Darling, try to understand. I'm here, right beside you.'

He had just returned from a 'respite care' stay in hospital and found it more and more disorienting.

We also got a little disoriented from these times. There was always, for example, the new selection of clothes. There seemed to be a general interchange in these places, although we did our best with name tapes.

Sometimes we rather liked the different things. I can remember a man's dressing gown I took quite a fancy to – the old, traditional 'checked' kind. We usually got most of the pink underpants back, however. I liked to think (since they obviously had to put some of the pants through their own laundry) that we may have been responsible for a pinkish tinge in quite a few other garments in the hospital – a cheering thought.

Once father came back without his teeth. I'm rather ashamed to say it took us almost twenty-four hours to notice that his upper plate was missing. He had always kept his false teeth in at night and, in recent days, we had to do a lot of persuading to get them out to clean. (Gone were the days of my light-hearted youth when I used the joke that 'you knew that you were in love with someone if you felt you could share a toothbrush'. These days I felt I could probably share the teeth if they would fit.) It was when he started on the breakfast toast next morning that we noticed he was having a problem.

We searched our bedroom and bathroom without success and came to the conclusion they must have been left at the hospital. From the response of the ward sister on the telephone, we gathered it was fairly common. She promised to 'look out for them'. (Where could they be? Decorating the mantelpiece?)

A couple of days passed and we had to keep father (who still enjoyed his food) on shepherds pie and porridge. We were really worried. There would be no way, short of giving him a general anaesthetic, that a mouth impression could be taken from him now for a new set.

Then – joy of joys – we heard from the hospital that a ward maid had found them when cleaning along the skirting board under the bed.

I drove twenty miles to collect them.

Another effect of the 'respite care' week was a succession of more disturbed nights. Gwen was incredible. Still sleeping in the big double bed, she was instantly awake if he started to get up, and ready to help him. I, along the passage with my bedroom door open, would hear the shuffle-shuffle of their progress to the loo, and would usually get up also. Father was getting weaker and his progress slower and more unsteady. We had been given a wheelchair, so he could have sat in the chair and been wheeled to the bathroom. But it was not possible without a long period of persuasion and pleading. He did not understand its use, and he was over six foot and still strong. So we helped him stagger along to the bathroom. The week after he had been away in hospital Gwen and I would do this every two hours.

I went on wondering what happened during these 'respite care weeks'. Who had come when he asked where Gwen was, and what had they said? Had he continually got out of his bed at night or were there rails to prevent him? How had he found the loo? What did they say or do at constantly wet sheets? This was something I never could bear to ask. The respite we were getting was saving our sanity and one of the 'suggestions' from professionals was that we neither visited nor asked much about the time he spent there. But it could not be denied that things were getting worse. He was slower and more unsteady, more easily irritated, needing more help for every simple action. How long could we go on?

We tried so hard to help him enjoy the things he used to like doing. He had been a pipe smoker all his life, and the action of filling the pipe was something he still did – only he filled it now with broken matches or anything else that was handy. I used to get the tobacco and fill it for him: even sit beside him and light it, puffing away at it until it 'drew' a little and then handing it to him. He would take it gladly, smiling, and give a weak puff or two – but did not go on.

Watching us from a distance, friends would say, 'I don't know how you and Gwen keep going, Rhena. You're marvellous.'

I can't speak for Gwen, but I kept going by holding fast to God's ready, outstretched hand. There were times when I would go to my room and stretch up my hands as high as they would go as if I would pull God down.

'Lord Jesus, come *here*. Help me. I need you!'

Twice a week I went swimming. It involved a drive of eighteen miles through the countryside to reach a good swimming pool, but it was important to me: an hour and a half of being alone with space around me. It was an effort to keep it in my programme, but worth it. I used to go on the days when father would get meals on wheels, which meant that we had no lunch to get and Gwen would have some company.

It was so easy to feel trapped. Here I was with a commitment to starting a new work in the UK and yet unable to leave Norfolk for a night, with no visible end to the situation. I wrote to my prayer partners:

Dear friends,

Being on 'standby' at an airport is a worrying business. Is there going to be room on the aircraft or not? Do you let the friends who brought you to the airport leave, or keep them there in case you have to go home again? How about your luggage? Will it be loaded onto the aircraft whether you go or not and how will you find it again if you don't make it on board?

But being on standby with God is different. I

am not the first of God's servants to be called to a
ministry only to find that there is a period of waiting involved... *(February 1991)*

But in my private prayer diary, a year later, I drew a
little picture of a figure laden with shopping bags and
walking around in a circle. Leading from one part of
the circle was an open door. I could look through it as
I passed. But across it was a firmly locked 'child's
gate' and I knew I couldn't go through.

This was my life – trapped in a seemingly eternal
circle. Now and again, I caught glimpses of what lay
somewhere in the future – the vision of 'Outlook'. I
used to explain it as 'a kind of Youth for Christ at the
other end of the scale' and avoided the term offered
me as a joke: 'Geriatrics for Jesus'! But there was no
way I could do more than look and pass on. The time
was not yet.

The struggles went on. We began to leave him
sometimes in dressing gown and pyjamas all day.
Previously we used to dress him. It seemed much
more dignified somehow. We noticed they always did
at the hospital, and he looked good when he came
back in his trousers and a jersey (often neither of them
his). But somehow the struggle to keep his trousers
clean got too much for us. Pyjamas were easier to
wash.

Persuading him to let me cut his nails was another
huge effort although he continued to shave himself if
the electric razor was put into his hand. (Learning
how to clean this was another acquired skill of those
days.)

But we laughed. Sometimes. Once he had a chest
infection and I had bought (under instruction) Friars

Balsam. It was, I was told, to be inhaled in hot water. I thought it rather unpleasant stuff, but duly brought a bowl of it to father and tried to explain what he should do.

'Take a deep breath over the bowl,' I said, demonstrating it, 'and then blow it out sideways.' I got quite nicely into a rhythm with the deep breath (horrid stuff!) and then the blow. Father, willing but confused, began to join in. Breath ... blow. Breath ... blow. I suppose it was entirely predictable that we both got out of step at the same time, took the deep breath at the side and blew strongly together into the bowl of hot water. It took ages to clean up the mess.

Evening services in our parish took place about three miles away, in a small and beautiful church surrounded by tall trees that reminded me sometimes of Africa. On Sunday evening I could sometimes get away: 'Lord, are you still there?'

The words of the hymns could calm me sometimes:

> In heavenly love abiding,
> No change my heart shall fear;
> And safe is such confiding,
> For nothing changes here...

How will father die? Will there be a rush of blood from the cancerous bowel? Will he die in his sleep so that Gwen wakes up to find him dead? Will there be a crumpled heap at the bottom of the stairs when I come home from this service because he tried to go upstairs and I wasn't there to help?

> The storm may roar without me,
> My heart may low be laid;

But God is round about me,
And can I be dismayed?

'Take a week at a time,' a kindly district nurse once said to me, 'and, if you can't manage that, try a day at a time.'

'Or an hour at a time,' I thought. 'I could make an hour.'

❧ CHAPTER TWELVE ❧

In early March I nearly lost the family cat. I had taken her to the vet and she escaped from the cat basket in the middle of Swaffham. I stared in horror as she streaked down the High Street. My first thought was that, if I lost her, father would miss her so much

I know we are not the first people to discover that family pets do relate to illness in the humans they belong to. Tigger, though in essence entirely selfish as are all cats, was a great comfort to father. She would spend most of the time curled up on his bed, and he often put his hand down to feel her. What would happen when he reached his hand for her now?

Meeting the traffic, Tigger swerved into the supermarket car park. Panting and distraught I followed her and viewed with alarm the fences around the car park. They led to people's gardens, other streets, waste ground, a local garage. No cat was in sight. Frantic enquiries from people brought no response and only, just as I was leaving the car park, a timid meow saved the situation. She was crouched under a car.

At least one crisis had been averted.

'I have to share with you,' I wrote to my African prayer partners later that month, 'that I am still delayed in my intention to move into full-time work with the elderly here in Britain. My father (92) remains in need of daily nursing care. So I am still operating the preliminary plans for 'Outlook' from an office/bedroom in my parents' house in Norfolk, waiting His time. Please pray with me that I demonstrate the spirit of peace, patience, and trust in the Lord during this waiting period...'

The Name of the Lord is a strong tower. The righteous runneth into it and is safe. *(Proverbs 18:10)*

I had seen that text painted on a wall in a church in Ethiopia at a time of great persecution and fear. It was a time when Ethiopian Christians learned to sing very quietly so as not to draw attention to themselves; when churches were being closed each week; and many leaders were in prison for their faith. Now I needed that 'strong tower'. And it was there.

Morning by morning I went into the 'spare' bedroom early and sat by the window as the sun rose over the low hills.

'Lord, this seems such a long wait ... I feel so weak...'

Perhaps most often in my mind was the question whether we should simply carry on until father died; or whether we should try to find a nursing home to take him before we reached the end of what we could do. He no longer really knew where he was. Was it time to consider finding somewhere else for him? How many of such homes took in patients with dementia? What did they charge? Could we bear to leave him somewhere? Would he become entirely confused once away from the still-familiar family home?

'Oh God, my father, King and Lord, lead me on.

Guide me for I delight to do Thy will...'

Letters from friends and others I did not know encouraged me.

'God will release you to do this work in His own time,' they would say.

' But when, Lord, when?'

I said 'When?' to the Lord. But I never said 'Why?'

I have met people since who torture themselves with that question. 'Why me, Lord? Why does it have to be my son (or daughter, or husband, or father) going through this? Why should it be me caught in this trap of caring?'

I don't know why I didn't ask that question. It wasn't because I was super-spiritual. It may have been that I recognised the experience as a preparation for the new ministry to which I knew I was called. But mostly, I think, it was because I recognise that we really should not ask God why.

'Who is this that darkens counsel by words without knowledge?' he demanded of the questioning Job. 'Where were you when I laid the foundation of the earth and determined its measurements? On what were its bases sunk, or who laid its cornerstone? ... Who shut in the sea with doors when it burst forth from the womb; when I made clouds its garment, and thick darkness its swaddling band?' (Job 38 – 42).

And Job was silenced and humbled. 'I know that Thou canst do all things, and that no purpose of Thine can be thwarted ... I have uttered what I did not understand, things too wonderful for me that I did not know...' (Job 42).

I was in a situation the Lord had led me into. I had followed him too long to start doubting him now. I would not question him.

The respite care continued at the Kings Lynn Unit. By April 1992, the doctor in charge there was beginning to accept father would soon not be able to be cared for at home, and some arrangement for permanent care would have to be considered. A session was set up in early May for Gwen and I to come to Kings Lynn and discuss the situation. I wrote to the Norfolk County Council for a list of homes and left for a conference in the Midlands.

The conference was the main BCMS conference in Swanwick. I remember it for the love and care showed to me there by friends of long standing. All those closely involved with overseas mission know that plans for the future are often delayed. Visas don't come through; children are sick; aircraft land where they shouldn't; 'permission' to start this or that work sometimes took years to be granted. Yes, missionaries and those close to them understand the word 'wait'. In addition, some of the mission supporters at the conference were elderly and had been in the same 'caring' situation that I was in now. I began to experience the kinship that there is among those who care for the old and terminally ill.

From this three-day conference in Derbyshire I went to address a lunch meeting in London under the banner of Christian Viewpoint. In a hotel dining room, to over a hundred ladies, I shared something of my testimony over the years in Africa and also mentioned my new calling from the Lord and the fact that, although I was in a waiting period, I was confident God would free me for it at the right time.

I remember two ladies afterwards looking at me with something approaching awe.

'I wish I had as much faith as you have,' one of

them said to me afterwards.

Faith. Did I have so much? What had Jesus said? 'If you have faith as small as a mustard seed, you can say to this mountain, "Move from here to there and it will move. Nothing will be impossible for you" ' (Matthew 17:20). I was once given a little bottle of mustard seeds. I still have them. They are so tiny. If one drops from my hand to the floor, I cannot find it again. Surely, at least, I could summon up that much faith!

I drove home up the M11 that same evening, into the quiet forests of Norfolk. Twenty minutes before I actually arrived, the hospital phoned Gwen. Father was sinking. He had a chest infection – pneumonia. 'The old man's friend'.

I had asked one of the doctors once, 'Why do people seem to die in the respite care weeks?'

He answered thoughtfully, 'I think sometimes people want to go, but when they are at home, surrounded by those that love them, who are meeting their needs and caring for them, they feel they must hold on. When it is quieter and they are more alone, they can quietly let go.'

We went to the hospital immediately. Father was breathing with difficulty. He was not conscious. Gwen and I stayed with him some hours, murmuring messages of love. He died that night.

It was difficult to imagine life without him.

Norfolk County Council had sent me a list of possible residential homes. I found it in the mail waiting for me, and laid it aside. Perhaps it would be useful in my new work.

How often I had said to others, 'I see Dad as he will be when this is over.' But in the weeks following his death I could only think of him as he was in those last years – trying so hard to live with the overwhelming fact that his mind was slowly dying.

In his book *My Journey into Alzheimer's*, Robert Davis wrote of his own death:

> Some day my heart will stop beating and my body will be coldly stretched out. Someone unknowingly will say, 'Bob Davis is dead.'
>
> I am not dead! At the moment my heart stops beating I will at last be fully alive.

At last father is 'fully alive'. What is he experiencing in heaven? Surely far more than any of us can dream of, for 'No eye has seen, no ear has heard, no mind has conceived what God has prepared for those who love him' (1 Corinthians 2:9).

I have been and done many things in my life. I have been known as a grammar school teacher, a missionary, a magazine editor, a lecturer in Communications, a writer, a Church Communications Officer, and, now, as the National Director of a new organisation. But I remember the words of an old ex-farmer in Norfolk who walked slowly and painfully (because of an arthritic hip) beside me on my way to church soon after my father's death.

'You were a good daughter to your father, Rhena,' he said. 'Yes, a good daughter.'

There are worse epitaphs.

❧ CHAPTER THIRTEEN ❧

I drive a lot and I suppose it is natural to me to see many things in terms of driving. For all of us there are 'waiting' periods in our lives, and I have often thought of these as temporary breakdowns in a main road 'parking bay' or on the hard shoulder of a motorway. Life in general is going on its normal way quite near us but we have stopped. The noise is phenomenal as cars, lorries, coaches and motor bikes all thunder by. People in different cars talk, laugh, quarrel, eat sweets, turn on the radio and talk on mobile phones, hardly giving us a glance. It is all the more frustrating if we had a clear destination and time-schedule in our minds. Just when is the AA going to arrive?! When can we get going again?

People who lose their jobs must feel like this. I understand that if you don't find work within six months, the likelihood of getting another job lessens. As the time in the lay-by lengthens, it becomes ever harder to rejoin the mainstream of life.

Looking back, I cared for father for just two years. Among the millions of carers today in the UK, this is a short time indeed. People can be in this situation for ten years, fifteen, even longer. None of us really knows when the caring situation will end. Those we care for may live much longer than the medical advisers thought they would; or they may suddenly die. When we are actually in the caring situation we have to force ourselves to stop watching the traffic and act as if this period will go on indefinitely, leaving it to God to bring it to an end when he wills.

However, the question does arise: could it be in the will of God that we ourselves should bring the period to an end? The 'just walk away' of the local GP did stay in my mind, not because a literal 'walking away' was ever a possibility, but because we are free individuals and can take action. Other people can help; there are homes available when we reach the end of our own abilities and strength. I remember writing about this long ago in the countryside of Africa when I saw missionaries putting up with situations which were beginning to destroy them and their family. God has given us a 'way of escape' when things become intolerable (1 Corinthians 10:13), and we have to recognise what that is and when to take it.

So at last it ends. The burden is lifted. But can we straighten up? What about the relief we feel now and the guilt that comes with it? How can we 'work through our grief' when it has been our daily companion? Can we remember how to relate normally to other people? Can we really sleep for six or seven hours at a stretch, or have we lost the habit for good? And, perhaps more importantly, do we still know where we want to go? I drew another picture in my prayer diary. The door in the circle was now open and I had paused in my walk around the circle, looking towards it, momentarily frozen in my tracks.

I think sometimes that the Bible is written for those who venture out for God. Jesus said, 'I am the light of the world. Whoever follows me will never walk in darkness, but will have the light of life' (John 8:12). Somehow, the idea of Jesus as a light had always been a static one. But now I saw it differently. It was on the move, and I had to follow it.

Where was the vision that God had given me? Could I find it again? It had to come off the back burner and become fully part of my life. A month after father died, I sat down again at the small home computer in my bedroom and looked back at some of the things I had written when this vision of taking the gospel of Christ to the over-60s had first come to me in the quietness of another land. I took out again the folder of letters I had received from older Christians in the UK. Over eighty people had written to me following my first article in a Christian magazine. I read some of them through again, glad that I had kept them:

'The need is very real ... older people feel out of it in these days when they feel unwanted...'

'I think it is a wonderful idea to encourage older Christians to minister to their own age group ... there does appear to be a general lack of love for the elderly, inside and outside the church...'

'There are two great clouds that descend on the over-60s: don't be too positive as an OAP and certainly crawl into a corner if you are a widow. People just don't want to know you or expect you to be able to do anything, and that's pretty dispiriting...'

Yes, the need was still there and so was the vision. The trouble was that it was time to stop dreaming and face reality. I was momentarily terrified. Start an organisation? How? And where should I begin?

Once more, Scripture came to my aid: 'You broaden the path beneath me, so that my ankles do not turn over' (Psalm 18:36). I looked back in my prayer diary at my sketch of the open door and me staring through it and I added a nice broad path in a red pen. 'OK, Lord. Here we go.'

I started talking to church leaders again. I remember two responses in particular.

'Do you think a woman could take up leadership like this in the UK church?' I asked one. (Remember I had been twenty-eight years in Africa).

'As long as it's children or old people, yes,' was the somewhat daunting reply. The fact that it actually was 'old people' didn't help.

The other occasion was when I was sitting by a young clergyman at a John Wimber conference. He asked me casually what I was doing and I poured out my heart to him about the vision I had.

'Hmm,' he said, looking me over. 'Yes. It's always a problem to know what to do with lady missionaries when they come back from the mission field.'

I spent time alone in my bedroom with my small computer, putting together a 'proposal' (for whom?) and in the evenings I tidied up the papers that had accumulated over the past months. Thus I saw a small hand-written note, nearly a year old, from a friend, saying he had met someone from Help The Aged in a train who might help me when I got started. A business card was attached.

I added the name on the business card to the rather small list of people-who-might-be-interested in the 'proposal' I was writing, and went to see if I could sign on for the dole since the Invalid Care Allowance had stopped and I was still under 60.

It turned out I wasn't eligible for unemployment benefit because the contributions paid for the last twenty-eight years by my mission society didn't cover it. I could apply for income support if I needed it.

For the moment I didn't, but I 'signed on' every fortnight to make sure my 'stamp' was paid. For the time being I stayed with Gwen in the family home.

My 'home-made' proposal for the starting of 'Outlook' was passed on, in the Help The Aged offices, to the Church Development Officer. He suggested we had a talk, which we did, and in the next day or two I received his letter dated 2 July 1992, just two months after father's death.

As requested I have been giving OUTLOOK a lot of prayerful thought. Before Help the Aged, or any other similar organisation for that matter, can give OUTLOOK serious consideration, it needs to be a formally constituted legal body – with constitution, officers, a bank account, etc. As an enabling charity I think it falls to us to see that this gets done. Consequently I have reserved Meeting Room 2 in our building for OUTLOOK's Inaugural AGM to be held at 5 pm on Monday 5th October 1992.

I think it was what is known as a 'kick start'.

On the 5 October, a small group of people (about twenty-five) met in an office of the Help The Aged building, and OUTLOOK was born. I felt 'launched' before I'd had time to inspect the ship.

I have added this little story to this book because I think the move back into the mainstream of life is important for any carer, whatever age they are. We have been tied for so long, getting through each day. We have been so desperately needed and, if we are not careful, we can stay in the bondage in which we have been living, frightened (as I was) to move out and on. This is where we need a partnership with God. We move forward and find, after all, that He is there, guiding and blessing us. The faith 'like a mustard seed' is still enough. It can not only keep us steady. It can lead us on.

The prophet Isaiah wrote of God's guidance:

> And your ears shall hear a word behind you, saying, 'This is the way, walk in it' when you turn to the right or when you turn to the left. *(Isaiah 30:21)*

It was one of the first verses in the Bible I ever learnt. But as I have from time to time, thought back to it over the years, I have realised that perhaps it means that movement and guidance go together. Perhaps we have to begin to turn before we hear His voice. God sometimes challenges inaction at a time of need. 'Stand up!' he said to the distressed and humiliated Joshua. 'What are you doing down on your face? Israel has sinned...' (Joshua 7:10–11). There were things needing to be done.

Well, there are 'things to be done' in this world of ours and, if you have been a carer, then you have been given a unique opportunity to see and feel the rising needs of people who are helpless and in need. For you have come close to the darkness that hovers near each one of us, and you have returned to 'tell the tale'.

Don't stand still. Go on.

❧ CHAPTER FOURTEEN ❧

It was perhaps a year after my father's death. I was holding a small seminar in the Midlands called 'Senile Dementia: how does the Christian cope?' There were about thirty people present from a number of different churches.

'Does anyone want to share anything?' I asked towards the end.

'I want to,' a man said, getting to his feet, tears in his eyes. 'My wife has been suffering from Alzheimer's for several years now and I've never told anyone. The other church people think she's just ill with arthritis or something.'

We listened as he told us a little more. How, at first, he and his teenage children had tried to pretend it wasn't happening and constantly 'covered up' for her. 'In the end, we just re-organised our lives around her,' he said, 'and we do that still, but we don't like to admit to anyone that she is mentally ill. Very few people know.'

My mind went back to that woman where I had delivered meals on wheels.

'Silly old fool!' she had said of her husband.

She did not really see her husband as a fool. It was a remark of embarrassment, of denial that anything except a little 'silliness' was wrong with him: a refusal to accept, or at least to admit to others, that he was ill.

Perhaps the first thing we have to do, if our lives touch those with Alzheimer's or senile dementia, is to see it as a disease (when it attacks young or middle-aged people) and as one of the possible consequences of getting into their eighties or nineties, for the old. We could also take an interest in, and perhaps support, those who are seeking a cure. To our non-medical eyes, it appears that parts of the brain are dying, just as any part of our exceedingly-complex body can begin to wither and die as we grow older. The term Alzheimer's is most frequently used when a much younger person experiences the same symptoms. In either case, the sufferer needs as much sympathy and gentleness as does any person we know who is ill. Refuse the attitudes others might have, and speak openly about it.

'How do you like living with a lunatic?' someone once said to me in a kind of angry grief at her own desperate situation.

Is this what caring for someone with dementia is? Living with a lunatic? Far from it. The person is still there, wrestling with the growing mists around them, needing someone there to touch them and say, 'You are not alone. We'll take this journey together.'

It is the same message given to anyone in the grip of a terminal disease. Whether it is the mind or the body that fails, common humanity must say, 'We're here. Hold on.' Why is it easier to say that to the sudden victim of a road accident than it is to an old man or woman suffering from senile dementia? People are still afraid of getting too involved with the mentally ill.

'I've got a lousy job,' someone on a district council

complained whose job was to find accommodation in the 'community' for those with psychiatric problems. 'Housing the nutters!'

This is the kind of careless attitude which greatly increases the strain laid upon those caring for the mentally ill within a family. It can make them feel ashamed, as if they must keep the sufferer out of sight if they are not to be whispered about in the local community.

'That's Mrs Jones, you know,' people say in a lowered voice in the post office queue. 'Her husband's – well, you know – not quite there. You know what Pam told me the other day. She was passing the house and there the old man was, peering out of the front door in just his pyjamas!'

There has been a lot done in recent years to alter attitudes to mental illness in general. People have learned to accept the odd behaviour of a group of children or young people who are brought in a bus to the swimming pool or the seaside. It is time the same friendly acceptance was given to those older people who, after a lifetime of normality and hard work, spend their last years in the mental darkness of dementia. To de-personalise, to reject, to despise any living human being is to, in some measure, dehumanise ourselves.

God himself looks upon the old with gentleness and compassion:

> Even to your old age and grey hairs I am he. I am he who will sustain you. I have made you and I will carry you... *(Isaiah 46:4)*

There are times in our human families when family

members gather and support one or another in a special time of need. In the Christian family too, I believe there are times when we should accept the responsibility membership of that wider family gives us, and care for certain of our members when the time comes that they need help.

Robert Davis gives a frightening picture, much worse than I have spoken of, of the terrors that can come even to Christians in the grip of Alzheimer's:

> Perhaps the first spiritual change I noticed was fear. I have never really known fear before. At night when it is total blackness, these absurd fears come. The comforting memories can't be reached. The mind-sustaining Bible verses are gone... I have to wonder if the ceaseless walking and wandering of Alzheimer's patients is their effort to raise themselves out of the agony of their own fears.

As in earlier days I saw my father wince and turn aside from the noise, confusion and violence on the TV, carelessly left on; as I saw him reach out so often for the reassurance of our presence, and experienced how I could calm his anxious mind by holding his hand and quietly praying for him, I knew that we need, as a Christian family, to help those who travel this particular road in today's society. Somewhere is the person or group of persons that God will speak to about this.

So what of the carer? He or she is not outside the boundaries of God's love. 'All nature grows in the dark' and it is in the dark times of life that we learn very special lessons of God's love and, incidentally, discover around us a fellowship of 'unsung heroes'.

I quote Robert Davis for the last time:

I never really knew how many people are in this special fellowship because I only looked into the lives of the heroic from my wholeness. Now I have walked through that door and find a great crowd of loving, suffering, unsung heroes who are courageously living with Christ through the fellowship of his suffering. Paul went through this door and, though he sought healing, Christ answered, 'My grace is sufficient…for my strength is made perfect in weakness' (2 Corinthians 12:9).

Over thirty years ago, as I set out for Africa I wrote some home-made prayer cards. They bore a message I still believe in:

My weakness: His strength.
My failure: His beginning.
My death: His life.

Rhena Taylor is now the National Director of Outlook, an organisation concerned with sharing the gospel with older people. Information is available from The Outlook Trust, 2 Hillview, North Pickenham, Norfolk PE37 8LA.

Information for patients and their families about Alzheimer's Disease is available from The Alzheimer's Disease Society, Gordon House, 10 Greencoat Place, London SW1P 1PH; telephone 0171 306 0606.

The Christian Council on Ageing (Epworth House, Stewart Street, Derby DE1 2EQ) run a dementia 'working group'. The group's aim is to create a network of concerned Christians in the field of caring for those with dementia, and to encourage a greater response from the churches in that area. Contact the Rev David Wainwright, 8 St Roberts Gardens, Knaresborough, N Yorkshire HG5 8EH.

OTHER TITLES FROM SCRIPTURE UNION

Closer to God: Practical help on your spiritual journey

Ian Bunting (ed)

We are all on a journey through life with God. For many it is a struggle. What may help us? In this book members of the Grove Spirituality Group write from personal experience and from their understanding of the way Christians have come closer to God down the centuries.

Dealing with death

Peter Cotterell

Death is often a taboo subject in our culture. This book takes a Christian perspective on the issues surrounding death, examines them in a practical way and looks at the question 'So why are we afraid?'

Heaven...It's not the end of the world

David Lawrence

By examining what the Bible does (and doesn't) say about heaven and eternal life, this book 'will challenge just about everything you thought you knew about heaven'.

'A clear and positive presentation of what appears to me to be the biblical viewpoint' (N T Wright, Dean of Lichfield).

Desert depths
Simon Parke

Jim, Tracey and Denis come to the desert in search of 'something'. This is Denis' account of their pilgrimage – one that challenges us to think about our own attitudes to God, to our faith and to other people.

How to pray when life hurts
Roy Lawrence

Prayer makes a difference because God makes a difference. Whether we feel guilty or angry, fearful or under pressure, this book offers practical help on how to pray when life hurts.

Make me a channel
Roy Lawrence

Many Christians struggle to be 'new people' in Christ, living 'life in its fullness'. Roy Lawrence argues that this is because we are not 'input/output' people. Without God's input, our good intentions flounder: yet if we don't share his gifts, we are not being the people he wants us to be. There are chapters on how we can receive and pass on forgiveness, kindness, love, healing, truth, freedom, hope, faith, joy, worldly possessions, Jesus and eternal life.

It makes sense
Stephen Gaukroger

A popular humorous and compelling look at the reason why it does make sense to be a Christian. Common arguments against faith are dismantled kindly, but firmly.

'This is the book to shove into someone's hand the second they become a Christian' (*Alpha* magazine).

So long, farewell and thanks for the church?
Morris Stuart
Why are previously committed and gifted Christians leaving the church, disillusioned and burned out? Inspiring and instructive, this book gives a biblical perspective on the mission of the church today.

Living with a purpose
Nigel Scotland
For Christians, life has an extra dimension. In society, in the church and in our relationships, God gives us a purpose in living. There are questions at the end of each chapter, for personal or small group use.

Making Jesus known: Scripture Union stories from around the world
Michael Hews
Scripture Union is active in 103 countries, spreading the good news to children, teens and adults. In this collection, fourteen staff members share some of their struggles – and tell us how they have seen God at work in their lives and ministries.

Mind over money
John Malham Bridges
A highly readable look at all aspects of money management from spending to saving, from giving to getting. A biblical perspective and a challenge to control money before it controls you!

Ready for God?
R T Kendall
God can turn up in many different ways and at unexpected times. Biblically based, full of real-life stories

and humour, **Ready for God?** encourages us to expect the unexpected.

Miracles
Michael Poole
Can we believe claims made today of miraculous healing? Answering this question and many others, Michael Poole show that there is no fundamental conflict between science and the miraculous.

Spiritual Encounter Guides
Stephen D and Jacalyn Eyre
A fresh approach to personal devotion for new or long-time Christians, the aim of these Bible studies is to help readers find intimacy with God. Titles are:

- **Abiding in Christ's love**
- **Sinking your roots in Christ**
- **Sitting at the feet of Jesus**
- **Waiting on the Lord**

Encounter with God
These books arise from popular series in the **Encounter with God** notes. Reworked and extended to book format, they retain the distinctive **Encounter with God** approach to the Bible. Titles are:

- **Encounter with God in Job** and **Encounter with God in Revelation**
  Dennis Lennon
- **Encounter with God in Hebrews**
  Joy Tetley
- **Encounter with God in 1 Corinthians**
  Morgan Derham